Modelling and Managing the Depressive Disorder
A Clinical Guide

This book will interest clinicians, researchers and inquiring readers. The authors argue that the current modelling of depressive disorders compromises research and clinical management and present an alternative approach to sub-typing and managing the mood disorders.

Prof Gordon Parker is Scientia Professor of Psychiatry at the University of New South Wales and Executive Director of the Black Dog Institute which is a research, clinical, education and training facility for mood disorders. He is an active researcher and, in 2003, was awarded a Citation Laureate for being the most highly cited Australian in the fields of Psychiatry and Psychology.

Assoc Prof Vijaya Manicavasagar is a Senior Clinical Psychologist with the Black Dog Institute, School of Psychiatry at the University of New South Wales. She has had a long-standing interest in the diagnosis and treatment of mood disorders from a psychological perspective.

Cover by **Matthew Johnstone**, Sydney-based artist and writer.

Modelling and Managing the **Depressive Disorders**

A Clinical Guide

Gordon Parker

Scientia Professor
University of New South Wales
Executive Director, Black Dog Institute
Sydney, Australia

Vijaya Manicavasagar

Director of Psychological Services
Black Dog Institute
Sydney, Australia

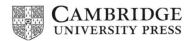
CAMBRIDGE
UNIVERSITY PRESS

CAMBRIDGE UNIVERSITY PRESS
Cambridge, New York, Melbourne, Madrid, Cape Town, Singapore, São Paulo

CAMBRIDGE UNIVERSITY PRESS
The Edinburgh Building, Cambridge CB2 2RU, UK

Published in the United States of America by Cambridge University Press, New York

www.cambridge.org
Information on this title: www.cambridge.org/9780521671446

© Cambridge University Press 2005

First published 2005
Reprinted 2006

Printed in the United Kingdom at the University Press, Cambridge

A record for this publication is available from the British Library

ISBN-13   978-0-521-67144-6 paperback
ISBN-10   0-521-67144-2 paperback

Every effort has been made in preparing this publication to provide accurate and
up-to-date information that is in accord with accepted standards and practice at the
time of publication. Nevertheless, the authors, editors and publisher can make no
warranties that the information contained herein is totally free from error, not least
because clinical standards are constantly changing through research and regulation.
The authors, editors and publisher therefore disclaim all liability for direct or
consequential damages resulting from the use of material contained in this
publication. Readers are strongly advised to pay careful attention to information
provided by the manufacturer of any drugs or equipment that they plan to use.

Contents

Acknowledgements

This book marks the culmination of a number of clinical research projects spanning several years and involving many of our colleagues at the Black Dog Institute. These include Psychiatrists Philip Mitchell, Kay Wilhelm, Marie-Paule Austin, Gin Malhi and our statistical adviser, Dusan Hadzi-Pavlovic, who are all co-Chief Investigators on our current National Health and Medical Research Council (NHMRC) Program Grant. Other key research staff involved in many of the studies considered in this book include Gemma Gladstone, Kay Parker, Joanna Crawford, Lucy Tully, Tania Perich, Therese Hilton, Gabbi Heruc, and Amanda Olley. In addition, we have been extremely appreciative of assistance from Christine Boyd, who has supervised data entry, and Yvonne Foy for preparation of this manuscript. We are particularly grateful for the cogent advice of Kerrie Eyers who commented on several drafts and helped us improve the book's 'readability', and to Kathryn Fletcher for editing assistance. We are also extremely appreciative of the creativity shown by the Sydney graphic artist, Aurah Wood, in capturing nuances of the 'psychotransmitter model' and creating personality 'icons'.

Much of our research was undertaken at the Mood Disorders Unit, a tertiary referral facility established in 1985, and which was incorporated into the Black Dog Institute in 2002. The Institute is based at Prince of Wales Hospital, housing a research team together with clinical services, education and training facilities, as well as a consumer and community resource centre, and allowing iteration between these components. This structure advances our long-standing model of seeking to have clinical observation inform research hypotheses and, in turn, research findings inform modifications to clinical practice as well as to education and training. Our web site (www.blackdoginstitute.org.au) provides additional information about the organisational structure and how research studies have historically evolved.

Our research would not have been able to be undertaken without long-standing support from Australia's NHMRC for funding our research over the last 15 years. We are also indebted to the Centre for Mental Health, NSW Department of Health, for providing Infrastructure Grant funding to enable research to be pursued actively. We are particularly appreciative of assistance from the many patients who have willingly allowed us to assess them in some detail for our research studies while undertaking their clinical assessment.

We thank Cambridge University Press' Richard Barling, Richard Marley, and Betty Fulford for their great assistance and professionalism in taking this project forward. We are also deeply grateful to our partners, Heather Brotchie and Stephen Mackie, for their patience and support.

Introduction

There are major problems in modelling the depressive disorders and in evaluating available treatments. In the last few decades, the Diagnostic and Statistical Manual of Mental Disorders (DSM) (American Psychiatric Association, 1994) model has dominated the classification of depression. It shares its largely dimensional model with the World Health Organisation's International Classification of Diseases (ICD-10) (World Health Organization, 1992) recent classificatory system. Thus, the current dominant model for conceptualising the depressive disorders is a dimensional or continuum view – with depression essentially seen as a single condition varying by severity.

We have long argued for a differing paradigm: one that allows (on the basis of specific clinical features) categorical status to certain expressions of depression such as melancholia and psychotic depression. However, once these more categorical conditions are excluded from the broad landscape of 'depressive disorders', there are difficulties in modelling the heterogeneous residue of non-melancholic conditions, as they are not categorical, vary in their status (as disorders, conditions, and stress responses) and are often multi-axial. For these, we favour a 'spectrum' model: viewing them as reflecting an interaction between salient life stresses and personality style.

In addition to challenging current diagnostic models we also challenge the 'evidence base' for evaluating antidepressant therapies. We question the reliability or 'gold standard' value offered by evidence-based approaches, at least as currently undertaken. We do not dispute the ideal – whereby judgements about the effectiveness of available antidepressant treatments benefit from randomised control trials (or RCTs) – when such data provide objective, impartial, systematic, and valid information. However, we note a number of intrinsic limitations to both the design and to the actual conduct of such trials and the 'meaninglessness' of the derived information. Many of the consequences include clinicians relying more on their own 'pattern analyses' rather than being able to trust results from the RCTs – a clearly unsatisfactory scenario.

Our alternative classificatory model allows that 'depression' can exist as a disease, a disorder, a syndrome and even as a 'normal reaction', and therefore requires a mix-and-match model for capturing both categorical and dimensional depressive disorders. Our model components are strongly weighted to clinical pattern analysis or what has been described by anthropologists as 'thick description', a base camp approach pursued by our team of clinical researchers before moving up the testing slopes of formal studies.

After establishing the Mood Disorders Unit in 1985, we spent nearly a decade seeking to distinguish psychotic and melancholic depression from the non-melancholic disorders. In the following decade, we have focused on developing the most appropriate model for conceptualising and differentiating the non-melancholic disorders from each other, with study results re-shaping our clinical approach to patients. Integral components of the model are tested in 'clinical effectiveness' studies, where we seek to define the most appropriate treatments for managing differing depressive disorders with increasing precision. We have cut our cloth on the iteration between clinical observation and research testing, and now we seek to persuade others to 'feel' its quality.

This book then reports a series of models and makes a number of treatment recommendations for managing the principal depressive conditions. As we considered melancholia and psychotic depression in considerable detail in a previous monograph (Parker & Hadzi-Pavlovic, 1996) this present volume gives greater attention to modelling and managing the non-melancholic disorders. We argue against an eclectic, and for a pluralistic approach to managing depressive conditions. This is best illustrated in regard to the non-melancholic disorders, where we seek to detail the impact of salient life events on predisposing personality styles, specifying the vulnerability points and arguing for pluralistic intervention strategies that we identify within our 'psychotransmitter model'. Thus, the book ranges from polemical to practical, and from provocative to precise. The identified models should not be seen as immutable, and we would welcome readers' responses, particularly if they could advance any of our current treatment strategies – and even coin a superior term to describe the 'non-melancholic' disorders.

The book is presented in four sections. Part I details the limitations to the current dimensional model for depressive disorders and the impact on clinical management. Part II considers the phenomenological definition and distinction of both *psychotic depression* and *melancholic depression*, and provides treatment recommendations based on published clinical effectiveness studies.

Part III & Part IV present our principal focus and aspirations for this book – how best to model and manage the non-melancholic depressive disorders. The 'diagnostic model' is rooted in clinical observation but, as noted, also respects a rich tradition of viewing these conditions as reflecting interactions between life events and vulnerable personality styles. The 'aetiological' model (termed a 'psychotransmission model') is partly metaphorical but, like all metaphors, seeks to advance communication – here, by identifying vulnerability processes for more rational pluralistic treatment approaches. At this stage, the 'evidence base' for the clinical effectiveness of the psychotransmitter model is not available beyond systematic clinical observation. We are currently testing its utility in 'real world' effectiveness studies, and we have some confidence in offering it as a logical model in managing these common conditions. Its logic emerges from combining the literature base with clinical observation, in avoiding therapeutic eclecticism (where a favoured therapy is applied non-specifically), and in promoting therapeutic pluralism in a commonsense and rational manner. We hope that readers judge it of value.

Gordon Parker
Vijaya Manicavasagar

The current model for depressive disorders and its impact on clinical management

A 'Declaration of Independence'

This book is provocative, deliberately so. It reflects frustration and disappointment at current modelling and consequently current treatments of depressive disorders. We will argue that conceptualising and modelling the depressive disorders along a dimensional continuum of severity has led to sterility of thought, clinical practice and research findings. It is time to make a 'Declaration of Independence'.

To paraphrase an address to the US Congress in 1776:

When in the course of human events, it becomes necessary to dissolve the dimensional view spuriously connecting one depressive condition with another, and to assume that separate or relatively independent conditions exist, a decent respect to the opinions of mankind requires that we should declare cause which impel us to argue for such separation.

We hold the following truths to be self-evident – that the depressive disorders are not all equal and that those endowed by their creator to enjoy the unalienable rights of life, liberty and the pursuit of happiness, are also entitled to a more sophisticated assessment and management model if they develop a depressive condition. We further declare that, as the current model of depression is destructive to that objective, it is the right of the people to expose its limitations, criticise it, and pour scorn on its quality of explanatory power. Prudence, indeed, dictates that DSM and ICD models long established should not be changed for light and transient causes but, all experience has shown, organisations are more disposed to continue, despite the associated sufferable nonsense, than to right themselves by abolishing the forms to which they have become accustomed. However, when a long train of conceptual poverty and management failures occur, it is our right, and it is our duty, to throw off such strictures and to provide new models for the individual patients and for the satisfaction of the therapist. We therefore appeal to readers to be absolved from all allegiance to an all-explanatory dimensional model, whether ideologically or politically developed, and to a greater confidence in and firmer reliance on a model allowing depressive conditions to be viewed as possessing relative independence from each other.

Having got the polemic off our chest, we will now proceed to argue key points in a manner somewhat more consistent with the academic tone of Cambridge University Press monographs, although every now and again we may move to a 'smoking' zone.

There has been an increasing tendency over the last few decades to view 'depression' as an 'it'. 'It' is then frequently interpreted according to the professional's particular paradigm. For instance, psychiatrists increasingly view 'it' as a disease reflecting a biochemical process and therefore likely to benefit from physical treatments such as antidepressant medication. Psychologists judge it to reflect schematic or attributional errors by the individual in viewing themselves, the world and their future, and therefore requiring cognitive behaviour therapy (CBT). To counsellors, 'it' reflects a disjunction between the individual and a range of social problems, and therefore benefiting from counselling and problem solving. The blind man's definition of the elephant springs to mind here. In practice, we currently have a situation where the professional background, training or disciplinary interests of the practitioner so shape the view of depression and its management that the depressed patient tends to be 'fitted' to the therapy rather than the therapy being shaped to respect nuances of the patient's particular depressive condition.

How has such confounding occurred? Let us document a few stages and a few markers along the road to obfuscation.

The wrong model

The current adherence to a dimensional model of 'depression', with conditions (if distinguished) differentiated largely on the basis of severity, has imposed a major limitation. Since the introduction of the third edition of the Diagnostic and Statistical Manual of Mental Disorders (DSM-III) (American Psychiatric Association, 1980), the North American model has viewed the depressive disorders as subdivided into 'major' and 'minor' disorders, and this division was extended by the formulation of less severe (e.g. 'sub-syndromal' and 'sub-clinical') expressions. Logically, how can a 'sub-clinical' expression have clinical status? The World Health Organisation's latest International Classification of Diseases, 10th edition (i.e. ICD-10) (World Health Organization, 1992) is also underpinned by a severity-based model, whereby depressive disorders are subdivided into 'severe', 'moderate', and 'mild'. Such models are variants of the former 'unitarian' model, which viewed depression as a single condition varying by severity. Both the DSM and ICD systems, largely by rejecting phenomenological definition and ignoring aetiology, use severity as the definitional marker, with the DSM system also dimensionalising duration and recurrence parameters.

As in any other medical field, any attempt to then create categories from dimensionally based data, risks producing pseudo-entities or pseudo-categories. This limitation is best exemplified in the DSM concept of 'major depression' (or 'clinical depression') as having diagnostic specificity and therefore being informative. As noted in our earlier monograph (Parker & Hadzi-Pavlovic, 1996), such a model has not generated replicable biological changes or correlates at a satisfactory level, and has not been informative in identifying treatment-specificity effects.

The last point is under-appreciated. Imagine for the moment that you are not a health professional reading this book, but an intelligent consumer who, after examining a list of DSM disorder criteria, realised that you had 'major depression'. You might wish to find out what might best 'work' for your condition. You might further want to know the evidence base for available treatments. Your reading is reassuring, at first. You are encouraged to find that psychiatry is no longer a sect-weighted field, but a *scientific discipline*, respecting an evidence base, and *weighting information* that comes from randomised control trial (RCT) studies – both evaluating treatments in comparison to each other and in comparison to placebo or control interventions. You are further reassured to learn that the database of RCT efficacy studies is the largest database existing in psychiatry, involving hundreds of thousands of subjects, and therefore capable of precise interpretation. You find that study parameters of improvement are standardised (e.g. a 'responder' is someone who has improved 50% or more over the trial period), so allowing differing studies to be compared against each other. In fact, you learn that such databases are so informative that they allow numerous explicit and authoritative sets of treatment guidelines to be generated in regard to the management of major depression.

The trouble with RCTs

But, when you look closer, you see empiricism without clothes. As noted in recent publications (Parker et al., 2003a; Parker, 2004), in reality the database is not particularly meaningful. Examples:

- One analysis of 'old' antidepressants (such as tricyclics) and new antidepressants (such as selective serotonin reuptake inhibitors, SSRIs) involving 150 studies and over 160,000 subjects returned a responder rate of 54% for each class (Williams et al., 2000).
- A more specific meta-analysis of 102 trials comparing only tricyclics and SSRIs found no difference in efficacy rates across these two classes (Anderson, 2000).
- A meta-analysis of psychotherapy trials compared to pharmacotherapy found only trivial superiority to pharmacotherapy (Robinson et al., 1990).

- Meta-analyses of nearly 30 RCTs comparing CBT, interpersonal psychotherapy and behaviour therapy reported responder rates of 50%, 52%, and 55%, respectively, suggesting comparable efficacy (DHHS Depression Guideline Panel, 1993).

In fact, when we look at responder rates in studies of antidepressant medication, psychotherapy, counselling, herbal treatment, and even bibliotherapy (i.e. reading books on depression), the responder rates are in the 50–55% range, suggesting comparable efficacy for all such strategies. Such non-specific results risk the cynical interpretation that All Roads Lead to Rome – or, at least that all treatments are equally potent in terms of managing 'major depression'. As noted by Holmes (2002), such results deliver the Dodo Bird verdict ('Everyone has won, and all must have prizes').

Such results could challenge our faith in RCTs and, as with religious agnosticism, there is the risk of abandoning religion merely because we have a problem with the local minister. The question here is whether the weighting to RCT-generated evidence is the obfuscating factor, or the procedures used in undertaking RCTs. We argue for the latter.

If we examine the RCT procedures for antidepressant drugs, the processes seem reasonable, on the surface. The study design procedures (and their voluminous documentation) appear rigorous, while their undertaking is presided over by august bodies such as the US Food and Drug Administration (FDA) who impose numerous procedures and strictures to ensure standardisation of measurement, evaluation, and the handling of those who withdraw or drop out. There is a sense of rigorous and hard science. The devil lies less in the detail however, and more in the aggregate because, if we keep our eye on the whole, then counter-intuitive findings can be explained.

A key finding is that if we examine the trajectory of improvement reported in FDA-supported studies of antidepressants compared to placebos, the difference in improvement rates is slight, at best. Two published analyses support that interpretation. In one study (Kirsch et al., 2002), the researchers examined the randomised control data for the six antidepressants approved by the FDA over the period 1987–1999 (i.e. citalopram, fluoxetine, nefazodone, paroxetine, sertraline, and venlafaxine). In the 47 trial data sets submitted to the FDA, there was no differential efficacy between the antidepressant and the placebo in nine studies while, for the remainder, the drug-placebo difference was two points on the Hamilton scale (Hamilton, 1960), which was interpreted by the researchers as 'very small and of questionable significance'. In another analysis of 52 pivotal FDA placebo-controlled studies of antidepressants (Khan et al., 2002), antidepressant efficacy was indistinguishable from placebo in 50% of the studies.

You may suggest that such results reflect a methodological limitation of meta-analysis and that, as the whole does not truly summate the parts, results would be different if individual studies were examined. However, if we turn to individual studies, similar counter-intuitive findings are evident. One is noteworthy – a study examining the efficacy of St John's Wort in comparison to both an SSRI and to placebo (Hypericum Depression Trial Study Group, 2002). Noteworthy, because the study design was impeccable (in terms of meeting, if not exceeding, standard FDA requirements). The sample was large (with a minimum cell size of 111 subjects), the study period (of 8 weeks) was sufficiently lengthy to address the particular research question, the study was overseen by several distinguished institutions, and the researchers comprised many of the most respected psychiatrists in North America. But the results? At the end of 8 weeks, the reduction in Hamilton depression scores was 27% for St John's Wort, 28% for placebo, and 29% for the SSRI, differences that are clearly trivial. The study is noteworthy in that its results are again counter-intuitive to common clinical opinion (where SSRIs are viewed as effective antidepressants, and St John's Wort judged as having minimal effectiveness for those with clinical disorders).

Consequences of non-specific findings

Regrettably, non-specific findings encourage some commentators to be highly critical of antidepressant drugs, claiming that such data demonstrate that they either act as placebos or are no more effective than placebos. The situation is not dissimilar for CBT. Despite its high scientific support and cachet value, when we examined (Parker et al., 2003b) the meta-analytic data set for CBT, we returned the Scottish verdict of 'not proven'. In essence, the data set could be interpreted as suggesting that CBT is no more efficacious than any other psychotherapy, counselling, or even placebo psychotherapy; but we suspect that such results more reflect CBT being tested as having universal application and according to limited RCT paradigms (with their emphasis on major depression, brief duration, and on measuring state depression levels). Non-specific findings are not limited to RCTs for 'major depression' however. Himmelhoch (2003) has described how RCT procedures for testing mood stabilisers such as lithium and valproate for bipolar disorder have also counter-intuitively failed to find differences between active drugs and placebo. Himmelhoch concluded (perhaps rather world wearily in relation to large scale, multicentre RCTs) that 'There is no treatment they cannot make equal to placebo.'

We suggest (Parker et al., 2003a) that there are two key reasons limiting the current capacity to interpret whether an antidepressant treatment is efficacious or not, be it a drug, a psychotherapy, or any other modality. Firstly, the use of constructs such as 'major depression' as a standard procedure in such studies. If 'major depression' is, in reality, a heterogeneous non-specific class comprising numerous depressive conditions, each with varying capacities to respond to differing interventions, then any condition–treatment specificity effects will be 'washed out' by homogenising disparate conditions under the 'major depression' rubric. Secondly, by testing treatments as if they have 'universal' (or non-specific) application, rather than as having specific benefits to certain conditions, there is again a diffusion effect. Thus, if a treatment is tested non-specifically against a non-specific condition, why should we not anticipate a meaningless non-specific result?

An analogy: if a woman develops a breast lump and seeks assistance, she is unlikely to be satisfied if the lump is defined in terms of its size (i.e. 'major', 'minor', or 'sub-syndromal'). In essence, she seeks more meaningful information (i.e. is it malignant or benign, does it require treatment, and what are the comparative advantages and disadvantages of differing treatments?). Let us imagine for the moment that breast lump research operated to the same parameters as occurs in the RCTs for testing an antidepressant treatment. Women with 'major lumps' (i.e. size counts, pathology ignored) would be assigned to receive any one of a number of treatments (e.g. radiotherapy, chemotherapy, radical surgery, and lumpectomy). If tested against an 'active' treatment applied non-specifically, differences might or might not emerge, depending on the mix of disorders. For instance, if a high percentage of the lumps were cancerous, we would anticipate that most of the treatments would be efficacious, but differentiation across treatments would be minimal. If most were benign (say, transient cysts), then the active treatments might have marginal efficacy at best, while their appropriateness (in terms of side effects) for those with benign conditions would raise major ethical concerns. Further, if the cysts had a high spontaneous remission rate, the capacity to demonstrate any truly effective treatment would be compromised. If, subsequently, several active treatments were examined across multiple studies using meta-analytic techniques (i.e. viewing each treatment as having universal application and with the mix of conditions and their pathology ignored), would we really anticipate clear differences emerging across the differing treatments? And, if they did, how could we interpret any such differences? Presumably, either that one treatment is universally more powerful than others, or that such differences more reflected the mix of disorders in the particular studies, and with one treatment being favoured only by a greater representation of conditions showing specific responsiveness to that therapy.

Medicine respects clinical description and diagnosis (particularly in identifying syndromes and classes), as well as the identification of causes and the pursuit of treatment-specificity effects. Such a model allows, for any defined condition, a gradient of effectiveness to be specified for differing treatments. Such a commonsense 'horses for courses' model does not currently underpin the conceptualisation and management of the depressive disorders, and we are all losers as a consequence. Clinicians have disinformation, while patients are further compromised by being at the end of a Chinese Whispers' information line. You may believe that the pharmaceutical industry is the big winner, but we are not so convinced. It must be frustrating (and expensive) for them to have to undertake multiple studies to obtain positive outcomes for licensing reasons, or to have to 'over-power' study numbers to begin to hope for a positive result, or in handling the recent controversies over the efficacy of the SSRI antidepressants. Some might argue that it is in the interests of the industry to have such a situation. This would hold if a pharmaceutical company had a drug (let us call it 'Nirvana') that has universal application. But, and at least up to the time of this book appearing, no such drug exists. The suggestion of the 1990s, that all antidepressant classes have similar effectiveness rates, is no longer believed by clinicians, or by the pharmaceutical industry. Any such claim or imputation has a limited shelf life, as clinicians are disappointed and frustrated by any over-sell. In the same way that most of us would welcome an antibiotic that cured all respiratory disorders, we recognise that certain antibiotics may be very useful for pneumonia, bronchitis, and other specific respiratory conditions but not always useful (and at times counter-productive) for other disorders (e.g. a pulmonary embolus). When antibiotics are used for relevant conditions, their 'usefulness rate' is increased beyond the rate observed when they are used indiscriminately, and their 'specificity' benefit becomes evident. As patients, we thus respect and benefit from the relevant application of those drugs. As clinicians, we appreciate knowing the 'rules of the game' for their prescription and knowing their right ecological niche (i.e. their rational and specific application). Both patients and clinicians, then bless the pharmaceutical company for having an effective product. As in the case of antibiotics, there is thus wisdom in knowing the specific circumstances for prescribing an antidepressant, including the advantages and disadvantages of using a narrow action or a broad action antidepressant drug.

Returning to the limitations of RCTs, there are other reasons why they (at least as the trials are currently undertaken) are delivering meaningless results. In essence, their theoretical advantages have been subverted by procedural components. Recruitment procedures are problematic and increasingly so. Most RCTs (of antidepressant drugs, at least) focus on recruiting relatively pristine subjects, in the sense that any such depressed individuals should not be suicidal, should not have any distinct co-morbid conditions (such as anxiety disorders, drug and alcohol problems, and personality disorders), while a focus on out-patients and volunteers generally excludes those with the more biological disorders such as melancholic depression. Thus, those taking part in studies generally bear little resemblance to depressed patients seen in clinical practice. Further, there is a high natural or spontaneous remission rate in those who take part in antidepressant drug trials, whether they receive the antidepressant drug or placebo. While it used to be in the order of 40%, it is now not uncommon for the responder rate to be 60% in many antidepressant drug trials, with Walsh et al. (2002) quantifying an increase in the responder rate (to both drug and to placebo) of 7% per decade. This suggests that confusion is possibly coming less from a perceived 'placebo response' in such studies and more as a consequence of many participants having either transient or ephemeral depressive conditions, and a high likelihood of a spontaneous remission shortly after baseline assessment. That is, studies are probably being increasingly weighted to those with more 'reactive' disorders who are likely to be primed to respond once the gun has been fired (i.e. received their first set of medication, be it drug or placebo). Thus, we suggest that the RCTs are failing us, in their application. End result, a meaningless database for clinical decision making.

In a recent article, the distinguished psychopharmacologist, Meltzer, observed, after noting several other problematic analyses, that the 'field would appear to have a lot of problems in its scientific basis' but that much of the negative results from studies 'represents the result of not taking all available information into account and a lack of understanding of the importance of specific features of the illness in question' (Meltzer, 2004). Precisely!

Treatment effects

The consequences of a meaningless database are predictable in creating an 'Everyone's a Loser and Everyone's a Winner' conclusion. The lack of differentiation of treatments invites the 'Everyone's a Loser' challenge, that all therapies act non-specifically or via a placebo effect, a rather demeaning interpretation for those with clinical disorders and a non-inspiring result for psychiatry and for current antidepressant treatments. By contrast, the non-specific database builds to the 'Everyone's a Winner' interpretation, as therapists can readily claim that *their* treatment is efficacious, whatever it actually is. This risks leading to what is described in literary criticism as the 'affective fallacy', where literature (here the therapy) is judged impressionistically rather than by any integral strengths. A hardly surprising consequence if integral strengths resist identification and definition as a consequence of the non-specific model of 'depression'. As noted earlier, this risks a procrustean model where the patient is fitted to the therapist's preferred treatment model – which may reflect the therapist's preferred style, disciplinary background, training or interest – rather than rational logic.

One could argue that this lack of differentiation of specific treatment effectiveness and the 'Everyone's a Winner' interpretation suggest that a single treatment for depression could be disseminated on a large scale at a population-based level. This might be analogous to treating all presentations of shortness of breath in the community with steroid-based inhalers. Whilst many would gain relief, others however (whose symptoms may be related to chronic infection) might actually worsen, while many would receive no benefit as the treatment was inappropriate. The 'average' patient in the community might be better off, but some individuals will be worse off. For the depressive disorders, where disability and suicide are key risks, some individuals will pay a very high price for receipt of a non-specific treatment.

We therefore argue strongly against a dimensional model of depression, the view that antidepressant therapies have universal application, and any model that ignores cause or aetiology. We understand the history, and the important watershed contribution of DSM-III. In the years prior to the development of DSM-III, North American psychiatry had lost its way somewhat, with an emphasis on Freudian psychodynamic treatments moving psychiatry further away from medicine, challenging the credibility of psychiatry and psychiatrists. As noted by Kirk and Kutchins (1992), the publication of DSM-III in 1980 'abruptly shifted emphasis from the aetiological psychodynamic perspective that had dominated psychiatry since World War II'. However, to replace psychodynamic causes with 'other' causes had certain risks. Rather than offend any one group, removing any consideration about aetiology or cause had pre-emptive benefits to the enterprise. In addition, there were 'integrative' models that minimised any logical need to consider cause. In 1973, Akiskal and McKinney had published an article in *Science* that was so influential that a variant was subsequently published in the *Archives of General Psychiatry* (Akiskal & McKinney,

1975). The model allowed that any number of disparate causes (i.e. genes, biological, and psychosocial factors, interlocking 'processes at chemical, experiential, and behavioural levels'), could effect changes along a 'final common pathway' in the diencephalon and thus cause 'depression'. If such a mechanistic process was valid, then the actual higher-order cause was effectively irrelevant, for here all roads converged on the pathway to Rome. Thus, a paradigm was born, weighting severity rather than seeking to distinguish types on the basis of distinctive clinical patterns, and thus minimising consideration of aetiology and phenomenology. Any differential impact on response to differing modalities was thus rendered more difficult to identify, while the expanding research endeavour would forever be compromised by the model or road map. But, why run, if you are on the wrong road?

At a theoretical level, 'depression' can be considered as akin to pain, at least at the symptom level. In the day-to-day practise of medicine, it would be rather unwise to merely prescribe an analgesic for pain and ignore its cause. It may be sufficient for a percentage of people who have transient and intrinsically self-remitting disorders, but not for everyone. A headache can be stress related, due to a toxin (e.g. too much alcohol), a disorder or syndrome symptom (e.g. migraine), or even a marker of a major disease (e.g. a sub-dural hemorrhage). Similarly, we suggest that depressive disorders may have multiple determinants and that there is little logical wisdom in ignoring identification of causes. Patients also want to know what has 'caused' their depression and, while an all-explanatory interpretation ('You have a chemical imbalance') may satisfy a percentage, most would find it too superficial. People seek to be informed as to *how* and *why* they (*as individuals*) have developed depression at that *particular time*.

Psychiatry, of course, has a rich history of aetiological speculation, but not necessarily a history that has commanded respect, with historical concepts such as humoral theories and more recent aetiological speculations such as 'masturbatory madness' among the more disconcerting. The early 20th century focus on psychoanalytic theory was perturbing, less because of the theories themselves and more as a consequence of their over-valued explanatory power. For example, for many clinicians, schizophrenia was a consequence of having a 'schizophrenogenic mother', with the possibility of schizophrenia being a biological disorder commonly dismissed or not even contemplated. As noted, the abandonment of aetiological formulation in the DSM-III manual was designed to put distance between the (medically weighted) new psychiatry and such fuzzy sect-based aetiological theorising, but medical disciplines usually progress better by testing aetiological formulations rather than ignoring them. So while we would intrinsically resist any aetiological theory that argued that 'depression' was necessarily caused by merely one of a set of multiple factors (e.g. parental experiences, early traumas, personality, coping style, abnormal hypothalamic–pituitary–adrenal (HPA) axis functioning, etc.), we suggest that the relevance of a range of psychological, social, and biological contributions does need to be considered when assessing any individual, rather than merely establishing that an individual meets 'caseness' criteria for 'major depression' ('it') and warrants the practitioner's preferred treatment modality.

Thus, in approaching the management of depression, we argue against a single-dimensional model and for one that respects the alternative possibility that 'depression' is not an 'it', that at the clinical level there are separate meaningful manifestations, that their causes are worthy of definition (for some shape the clinical picture and relate to the most appropriate treatment modality) and that no one therapy is likely to have universal application. In arguing for a 'sub-typing' model, we are not arguing for eclecticism, whereby you merely choose the model on the basis that it pleases you, but for pluralism, respecting that multiple parameters need to be considered in determining an overall explanatory model. We are 'splitters' rather than 'lumpers', looking for clinically meaningful cleavages (reflecting cause and clinical pattern) that have some level of treatment specificity. We are aware that truly independent 'types' are likely to be rare and accept that a sub-typing model has to constrain interdependent conditions as well as independent ones.

This chapter has attempted to identify the key issues that need to be conceptualised and considered before management can begin. Clearly, we have been critical and provocative. The reader can anticipate a more positive tone in the following chapters and that is easy, with some analogies in Chapter 3 suggesting that the problems noted here are not unique to psychiatry. However, if the current model is to be abandoned, how is it to be replaced? That task is less easy.

2

Defining and diagnosing depression

As much as it is important to know what 'depression' is, it is equally important to recognise what it is not. We suggest that '*depression*' (across the spectrum of its manifestations) is most directly captured by three features:
(i)   a depressed mood,
(ii)   a lowering of self-esteem or self-worth, and
(iii) an increase in self-criticism.

Phenomenologically, this weighting distinguishes 'depression' from *anxiety* (which is most commonly experienced as a sense of uncertainty, apprehension, insecurity, and fear, as well as hyperarousal (which can then lead to appetite and sleep changes). In *grief*, something of value to the individual (e.g. a partner, an ideal) is lost, but, in pure instances, the individual's self-esteem is not reduced (only in about one-third of grieving individuals does 'depression', with its associated drop in self-esteem feature, develop). As depression and anxiety (in particular) commonly co-exist (with the presence of each increasing the occurrence of the other), many clinicians are tempted to view anxiety and depression as synonymous. We also suggest that the phenomenological distinction of grief from depression is important, particularly in prioritising treatment strategies.

Distinguishing meaningful expressions of 'depression' is a less clear-cut process, but the obvious first task here is to contemplate what might distinguish '*normal depression*' and '*clinical depression*'. Normal fluctuations in mood, even if they distress us, are appropriate, and may even be desirable. To feel 'alive' is to think, feel, and react both to our environment and to the people around us. When we stop thinking, feeling, and reacting, we become like automatons or robots. When asked, more than 90% of people in the community have had episodes of 'depression' – defined as 'a depressed mood, lowered self-esteem and feeling hopeless, helpless, and pessimistic about the future'. Most report that such states only last minutes to several days. Such 'feeling blue' states can then be described as 'normal depression', allowing that depression can be a normal reaction to the vicissitudes of everyday life.

A depressed mood can exist on its own, or, if accompanied by a number of concomitant features (see shortly), be defined as a syndrome. Such a state (e.g. feeling 'depressed', not sleeping well, and experiencing other mood-state concomitants) does not, of necessity, establish 'disorder' status. For 'depression' to be a disorder, it not only has to have some level of severity, but it must also be persistent and impair function. Operationalising each of those parameters is less clear-cut. 'Persistence' (of at least 2 weeks) is formalised in systems such as the Diagnostic and Statistical Manual of Mental Disorders (DSM-IV) (American Psychiatric Association, 1994) and appears (in practice) to be useful, in that 'normal depression' usually lasts minutes to days. 'Impairment' should generally be interpreted in a commonsense way, in that the individual should have greater difficulty in engaging in tasks at work or at home. Attempts to distinguish 'normal' and 'clinical' depression across other parameters, including severity, are more difficult as depressed mood severity (like pain severity) is very dependent on the subjective attributional style of the individual.

As indicated, for most people, an episode of 'normal depression' (whether mild or severe) is relatively brief. It comes to an end either because it is destined to remit spontaneously and rapidly, or because the individual implements restitutive coping repertoires (e.g. discussing issues with and receiving support from friends, seeking distraction in work or hobbies) that serve to restore mental equilibrium. Although many clinically depressed people also engage in such behaviours, relief from depression tends only to be brief or superficial. Thus, the distinction of clinical depression on the basis of differing 'coping repertoires' is unhelpful, as coping secondary to the depression reflects a range of contributing factors. Similarly, differences in stressors or stressor severity are not particularly helpful in defining clinical depression. For every event or enormity that can occur in life which might trigger an episode of clinical depression, there will be people in the community who do not develop depression in response to that event, or, if they do become depressed, experience a rapid remission.

Clinical depression

As noted, a key feature to clinical depression is failure to experience a spontaneous remission. Why? We argue that, for those who have the more 'biological' types of depression, such a state is sustained and maintained by perturbed biological processes, while for those who have non-melancholic disorders, it is more their personality style and social factors that maintain the condition. Thus, while understanding what separates those who are 'vulnerable' (i.e. who develop 'clinical depression') from those who are 'resilient' to developing depression, it is equally important to contemplate why the clinically depressed individual has failed to experience a spontaneous remission. Distinguishing between factors which act as risks to onset of depression from factors that prevent remission of depression are issues of paramount importance to clinicians and are pursued in this book.

'Clinical depression' is predictably more severe than 'normal depression', with mood expressions including suicidal preoccupations as well as somatic features (such as sleep disturbance or poor concentration) being prominent. Our clinical descriptions do not convey fully the sheer range and depth of problems encountered by sufferers, who consistently report that it can be one of the most devastating events that anyone can experience. Authors who have been afflicted use descriptors such as 'a black hole' or 'dark shadow'. Other terms (such as 'black night of the soul', 'agony of mind or spirit', and 'anguish of the soul') reflect the inner turmoil accompanying the more biological clinical depressive disorders, often despite a lack of outward signs. While all depressive conditions are ultimately disorders of mood and loss of pleasure, many expressions encapsulate feelings of despair, wretchedness, and misery that obliterate all hope for recovery. It is no wonder then that people refer to their 'battle with depression' when describing their rehabilitation from a depressive episode.

Clinical depression is also a disorder of motivation, reflected in an inability to initiate purposeful activity, and to recover from everyday life stressors. Clinically depressed patients often suffer from lassitude and apathy, accompanied by or oscillating with overwhelming feelings of regret and guilt. By the time a diagnosis of clinical depression is made, most sufferers have repeatedly encountered numerous unsuccessful attempts at starting or trying to complete tasks that they would otherwise be capable of accomplishing. As clinical depression erodes a person's capacity to give and receive affection, it eats into the sense of 'connection' with others, leaving the sufferer feeling simultaneously abandoned, isolated, and discomforted by an enforced sense of solitude. As episodes are commonly recurrent, with sudden or insidious onsets, and lasting weeks to years, a progressively erosive process may, in itself, change the way an individual relates to others, perceives the world, and reacts to stress.

Clinical depression can go through many phases. Its onset may follow a period of anxiety and stress. Once established, it may plateau, or vary across the days and weeks. Improvement may be partial (termed 'remission') or complete ('recovery'), and further episodes can occur when the individual has only partially improved ('relapse') or following a depression-free interval ('recurrence'). Patients can present at any time during such cycles, perhaps most commonly when they are at their worst or after some improvement when they have regained enough energy to seek help. In the latter phase, they are often primed to experience benefit from appropriate management.

The formal presence of clinical depression can be estimated in several ways. As noted earlier, both DSM-IV and the International Classification of Diseases, 10th edition (ICD-10) (World Health Organization, 1992) focus on the severity, duration, persistence, and recurrence of depressive symptoms, with the presence of such features used to assign an overall diagnosis of (say) 'major' or 'minor' depression (DSM model), or 'mild', 'moderate', or 'severe' depression (ICD-10). In order to meet a diagnosis of clinical depression under the current DSM-IV classification, an individual would have to fulfil the criteria of five or more symptoms (listed below), with at least one having to be either depressed mood and/or loss of interest or pleasure. In addition, this state would need to last for more days than not over at least a 2-week period and be accompanied by significant impairments in social and/or work functioning. Other symptoms include:

• weight loss or weight gain,
• insomnia or hypersomnia,
• psychomotor retardation or agitation,
• recurrent thoughts of death or suicidal ideation,
• fatigue or loss of energy,
• feelings of worthlessness or guilt, and
• poor concentration or indecisiveness.

A similar criteria-based approach allows other DSM diagnoses to be made (e.g. major depression with melancholic features and dysthymia). Such criteria sets are useful in establishing a shared lexicon for superficial clinical communication but, as noted earlier, lack the precision necessary to advance clinical decision-making and research.

Depression can also be assessed by use of any number of scales, a dimensional approach that is compatible with the dimensional model of depression, with cut-off scores used to estimate the likelihood of clinical depression. However, most measures do not have a recommended cut-off, as the imposition of a cut-off score is necessarily imprecise (in generating both 'false positives' and 'false negatives'). Our 10-item screening measure for depression (the DMI-10) (Parker et al., 2002a) which is described in Appendix 1 has a cut-off of 9 or more. The cut-off has high sensitivity (in detecting those with 'true' clinical depression), but only moderate specificity (in that scores above the cut-off are returned by many individuals who are not clinically depressed). This is not inappropriate for a screening measure (where the aim is to select out those who are most eligible for refined assessment), and we therefore require duration (i.e. more than 2 weeks) and mood-related impairment criteria to be present, in addition to exceeding the DMI-10 cut-off, for considering the probability of clinical depression.

Clinical assessment of the possibility of a depressive disorder can be structured in multiple ways. We tend to employ a hierarchical approach, determining the likelihood of depression first:

(i)   Are you depressed?

(ii)   Has there been any change in your self-esteem or sense of self-worth?

(iii)   Are you being any more self-critical or tough on yourself?

Secondary questions to positive responses then probe mood state items such as feeling hopeless, helpless, pessimistic about the future, feeling like giving up, loss of interest, guilt, suicidal ideation and plans, and inability to look forward to things. Tertiary questions pursue domains that have the potential to assist diagnostic sub-typing, and include:

- Vegetative items such as appetite or sleep changes (increases or decreases).
- Diurnal variation in mood and energy (whether such features are worse in mornings, evenings, or unvarying across the day).
- 'Psychomotor disturbance' or PMD – best observed (the patient may walk slowly, have little 'light in the eyes') or admit to retardation and/or agitation as well as distinct concentration problems, and acknowledge great difficulty in doing basic things such as getting out of bed to bathe. The utility of PMD as a marker of melancholic and psychotic depression is explored in detail in other chapters. The development of our CORE measure of observable PMD is described in Appendix 2.
- 'Psychotic features' such as delusions, over-valued ideas, and/or hallucinations.

As noted earlier, a diagnosis of clinical depression is supported by a depressed mood with a reasonable number of associated features, present for at least 2 weeks, and associated with impairment in functioning (whether at home or at work). Once diagnosed, the 'type' of depression (i.e. psychotic, melancholic, or non-melancholic) and lifetime polarity (i.e. bipolar or unipolar) need to be established. We have noted above some of the features that have specificity to the psychotic and melancholic sub-types, and will consider their specific relevance in greater detail in Chapter 3. Bipolar disorder is often undetected at clinical interview, most commonly because the patient fails to nominate any features of 'highs', because probe questions are not asked, or because the clinician sets high thresholds (i.e. symptom numbers, duration of the 'high') for a positive diagnosis. Useful questions to screen for the possibility of bipolar disorder are:

- Do you have times when you feel 'wired' or energised more than usual?
- Do you then talk more and talk over people?
- Do you then spend more money and buy things you don't really need?
- Do you then need less sleep but not feel tired?
- Does your libido increase at such times?
- Do you then dress more colourfully?
- Do you then say or do things that you later regret?

If several bipolar disorder screen or probe questions are acknowledged, further questions should be asked assessing changes in creativity, self-confidence, things having 'special meanings', 'feeling special connections to people', 'things being very vivid and crystal clear', being impatient and irritable, and being more disinhibited. The possibility of true bipolar disorder is enhanced by such changes being observable to others who know the patient well (but this is not a mandatory feature), by such states coming on at a certain age (rather than being enduring, like a personality style, although bipolar disorder in childhood is recognised) and by the presence of psychotic features during such episodes, although the last is clearly not mandatory. We do not find episode duration to be of distinct diagnostic assistance, having managed patients whom we judged to have true mania, and who reported episodes as brief as 30 min and as long as 30 years.

Distinction of bipolar I and II is of clinical importance in that the drug management recommendations for each may differ distinctly. Bipolar I status tends to be occupied by those who have psychotic episodes and/or who require hospitalisation and/or those who have longer episodes clearly impairing their function. Drawing the boundary for those with bipolar II disorder, particularly in terms of distinguishing it from a normal personality style, is more problematic but attempted by our website-based (blackdoginstitute.org.au) self-test for bipolar disorder.

Any assessment of clinical depression clearly involves inquiring into a wide range of domains, including family history, early development, background medical, psychological and social factors (whether predispositional or not), proximal and distal stressors, previous treatments (and their usefulness), risk of self-injury and self-harm, current medications, compliance with previous treatments, response to previous therapies and therapists, and assessment of personality style. Apart from documentation and learning the particular individual's 'life story', the objective should be to develop a formulation explaining *why this particular individual is depressed at this particular time*. We believe that it is useful to provide a patient with a diagnosis and a 'workable' formulation immediately after their initial assessment, expressed with appropriate confidence and caveats, and with a recommended treatment plan formulated. The last is of deceptive importance in suggesting to the patient that there is a recommended strategy to assist them. Most usually, this is directed at resolving a current depressive episode, with consideration of relapse prevention usually best dealt with when episode remission has been achieved.

3

Depression sub-typing: independence and interdependence

'Taxonomy is described sometimes as a science and sometimes as an art, but really it's a battleground'.

– Bill Bryson (2003, p. 319)

The expatriate Australian psychiatrist, Barney Carroll, wrote that to understand depression is to understand psychiatry (Carroll, 1989). 'Depression' presents the greatest challenges and the greatest risk of hubris. It is a fantasy to imagine that a clear-cut typology either exists or can be readily derived, and the road to that castle is littered with numerous classificatory systems, variably proposed by observant clinicians and/or opinionated academics. The opinionated are now regressed to the mean by Consensus Committee processes, a theoretically constructive strategy but one that is disappointing in practice because of their reliance on formal evidence-based data while their risk-free ambience tends to reify the orthodox.

The previous chapter considered how 'clinical depression' can be defined, differentiated (phenomenologically from grief and anxiety), and diagnosed – all relatively straightforward issues in comparison to this chapter's domain. Here we seek to tackle a more difficult task: considering whether meaningful depressive disorders can be differentiated or cleaved from each other, whether such differentiation is absolute or a matter of degree (i.e. independence or interdependence), and then present a differentiated model of 'meaningful' depressive conditions which, we argue, allows differential treatment approaches to be provided on a more rational basis.

It is in our nature as human beings to seek simple models to assist us through life and, if a simple taxonomy did have explanatory power, we would all be most appreciative. However, rather than recognise that the depressive disorders resist ready understanding and modelling, we have tended in psychiatry to impose single models on complex data sets, in an attempt to make explicable (in terms of having a system and 'diagnoses') the inexplicable. We can also be too defensive in psychiatry, perhaps arguing that we lack a laboratory test or another gold standard, and therefore that the current 'system' is merely temporary until the gold-plated cargo arrives. Further, we have a tendency to believe that classification is more straightforward for all other disciplines, because the rules of the universe (unshared with psychiatry) allow more ready categorisation. Thus, in this chapter and elsewhere (Parker, 2005), we suggest that psychiatry is not unique, and make comparison with the fields of botany and palaeontology, quoting selectively from Bryson's (2003) '*A Short History of Nearly Everything*'.

But first, a history of attempts to classify depression, albeit short and selective as there are many excellent accounts (e.g. Lewis, 1931; Jackson, 1986). Dominant models can be succinctly encapsulated as (i) binary, (ii) unitary, and (iii) other. The binary view (two types) has a respectable tradition, including Old Testament documentation. For instance, Altschule (1967) suggested that St Paul (Corinthians 7: 10) distinguished between those depressions that came 'from God' (being otherwise inexplicable) and those 'of the world' (and so viewed as accountable by life stresses). This model was encapsulated in the 'endogenous/melancholic' versus 'neurotic/reactive' model of the 20th century, with the 'biological type' of depression being termed 'endogenous' as it emerged without any clear-cut determining trigger, in contrast to the other depressive 'type' ('reactive'), where life events were viewed as causative alone or as triggers to depression in a vulnerable individual. This longstanding dichotomous model was no longer sustainable when tested empirically. Numerous studies (including Mitchell et al., 2003) showed that life event stressors are only somewhat less likely to be experienced by those developing melancholic depression than for those developing non-melancholic disorders. Perhaps more importantly, we came to appreciate that life event stressors can quite commonly precipitate an episode of melancholic depression, particularly its first few occurrences, albeit with subsequent episodes becoming more autonomous and independent of distinct antecedent stressors. However, the lack of specificity of the risk factor means that any model which attempts to subdivide the depressive conditions on the basis of the presence or absence of such stressors is likely to have intrinsic, logical and practical limitations. Exit the concept of 'endogenous depression'.

The unitary view was stimulated, at least in the 20th century, by the British psychiatrist Mapother claiming that the binary distinction failed to demonstrate any differences at the level of cause, prognosis, and treatment specificity or differentiation, and that differences must therefore reflect gradations between conditions most commonly of disorder severity (Mapother,

1926). As we have previously noted (Parker & Hadzi-Pavlovic, 1996), multi-variate statistics failed to deliver support for the binary model, although we argued that this reflected the use of inappropriate analytic strategies (e.g. factor analysis) and by failure to include or appropriately measure the truly distinguishing clinical features. By then 'swamping' the truly differentiating clinical features (by including numerous non-differentiating items), true bimodality or a 'point of cleavage' was effectively prevented from being demonstrated. Thus, failure to demonstrate *clear-cut evidence* for a binary clinical feature model caused a retreat to a simpler unitary model.

We suggest that the expectations set for a precise binary model were unrealistic, in that it was unwise to expect the precision of a Linnaean botanical binomial taxonomy. Intriguingly, pre-Linnaeus, botany also had a 'highly whimsical' classificatory system. 'Animals might be categorized by whether they were wild or domesticated, terrestrial or aquatic, *large or small ...*' (Bryson, 2003, pp. 316–317, our italics). However, as Bryson notes, 'Even to-day there is more disorder in the system than most people realize' (p. 319), with the estimates of the number of phyla ranging from the low twenties to high eighties, and dependent on whether the biologists are lumpers or splitters. Bryson again – 'In principle, you ought to be able to go to experts in each area of specialization, ask how many species there are in their fields, then add the totals. Many people have in fact done so. The problem is that seldom do any two come up with matching figures' (p. 321).

Our capacity to develop a taxonomy might be thought to be closer to palaeontology than to botany, although the 'missing link' for the depressive disorders may be more conceptual than corporeal. While many believe that the processes for distinguishing apes from humans, and importantly the intervening 'missing links', establish clear-cut classes (e.g. *Homo erectus*, *Homo sapiens*), the Hominid genera actually have quite imprecise and blurred boundaries. Turning to Bryson (2003) again, by the 1950s, 'the number of named hominid types has risen to comfortably over a hundred', but in 1960 E. Clark Howell 'proposed cutting the number of genera to just two: *Australopithecus* and *Homo*' (pp. 388–389). Such a process is evident also in examining the classification of the depressive disorders, with phenomenological description (particularly by European psychiatrists) generating more and more putative sub-types, followed by a reductionist move to a binary (e.g. 'endogenous versus reactive') typology. Remember Benchley's observation, that there are two classes of people: those who divide the people in the world into two classes and those who do not (just as there are also three types of psychiatric researchers, those who understand numbers and those who do not). Bryson informs us about palaeontology currently: 'Altogether, some twenty types of hominid are recognized in the literature today. Unfortunately, almost no two experts recognize the same twenty', and 'The only way a name becomes accepted is by consensus, and there is often very little of that' (p. 389).

We suggest that the task involved in modelling 'depression' is more akin to interpretive anthropology where respect for 'thick description' is given, and where Geertz (1975) has suggested that its progress as a science 'is marked less by a perfection of consensus than by a refinement of debate'. Regrettably, the taxonomy of depression currently holds a sterile consensus position and is distinguished by a lack of a debate.

Perhaps the greatest limitation to determining how to model the depressive disorders is the assumption that any one model is explanatory. If, in reality and as noted earlier, 'depression' can exist as a disease, as a disorder, as a syndrome, as a normal mood state, and as an existential position, it would be unwise to consider that any single model (categorical or dimensional) is likely to have sufficient explanatory power. This is the position that we have arrived at in research that we have undertaken at the Mood Disorders Unit (Black Dog Institute) over the last few decades. We have progressively developed a hierarchical model, which assumes some categorical and quintessentially biological depressive conditions (i.e. psychotic depression and melancholia) and which we have sought to distinguish, from each other and from residual depressive conditions, on the basis of clinical features. For the remaining (i.e. 'residual') and heterogeneous conditions, we favour a dimensional model comprising key contributions from personality style and life event stressors contributing to the clinical 'pattern'.

The overall hierarchical model is illustrated in Fig. 3.1. The model assumes three classes: psychotic depression, melancholic depression, and a heterogeneous residual class of non-melancholic disorders. In all three, there is a mood disorder component (as all three are depressive conditions) and, while it may be true that the severity of depression increases as one proceeds from the non-melancholic to the melancholic and psychotic disorders, we argue against mood severity being used in any attempt to separate the classes (as a depressed mood is ubiquitous across classes). In distinguishing melancholic from the non-melancholic depression, we have argued (Parker & Hadzi-Pavlovic, 1996) for the observable presence of psychomotor disturbance (PMD) as a specific marker, with the PMD (involving a central cognitive processing difficulty, together with motoric retardation and/or agitation) being the surface (or recordable) marker of an underlying neuropathological process. An analogy can be made to certain neurological diseases, such as Parkinson's disease, where certain signs are diagnostic.

Fig. 3.1 Our structural model of three principal depressive sub-types.

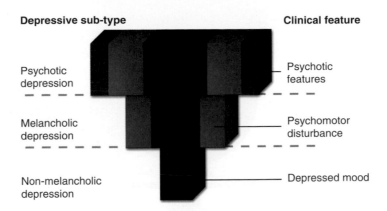

Depressive sub-type   Clinical feature

Psychotic   Psychotic
depression   features

Melancholic   Psychomotor
depression   disturbance

Non-melancholic   Depressed mood
depression

As one proceeds from melancholic to psychotic depression, PMD is generally more severe but, more importantly, there is now another class-specific clinical marker (i.e. psychotic features such as delusions, hallucinations, and/or over-valued ideas) that distinguishes psychotic from melancholic depression.

We suggest (with disappointment) that the residual 'class' of non-melancholic disorders lacks any specific defining clinical feature. The features of 'neurotic' and 'reactive' depression that have been suggested previously (such as reactive mood, or mood and energy worsening in the evening) are not 'positive' defining ones, more having obverse status, in essence informing us that certain features of psychotic and melancholic depression (i.e. non-reactive mood, mood and energy worsening in the morning) are absent. We are then left with the problem as to how to constrain such heterogeneity within the non-melancholic class. The Diagnostic and Statistical Manual of Mental Disorders (DSM) and International Classification of Diseases (ICD) approaches favour distinguishing disorders on the basis of severity, duration, or persistence and recurrence of episodes. We, however, argue for a model that seeks to prioritise two aetiological domains – life event stress (and particularly its meaning to the individual) and the individual's personality or temperament style – acting on a third and central component, the individual's self-esteem. As each domain is intrinsically dimensional, independent sub-sets of conditions are unlikely to exist, creating a predictable problem of determining the most clinically meaningful number of conditions. We suggest, having drawn analogies to the putatively 'firmer' fields of botany and palaeontology, that this task is not unique to psychiatry and that we should not therefore be discouraged if a pristine solution is not immediately available.

It may also be of concern that the hierarchical model moves from definition by 'clinical feature' specificity to definition by 'aetiology', as we proceed

Fig. 3.2 Our spectrum model of non-melancholic depression linking personality style with clinical symptoms, as illustrated for three expressions.

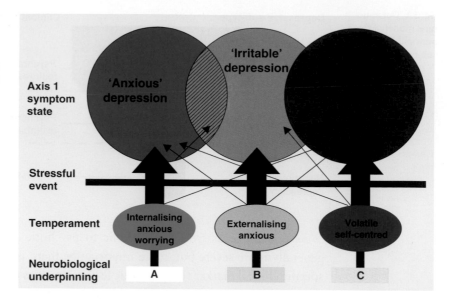

from the melancholic to non-melancholic disorders. However, for the non-melancholic disorders, we consider clinical features as having no more than a 'fuzzy set' potential in their capacity to differentiate, and therefore only consider their possible contribution to definition as a 'downstream' component. However, we do fish downstream, also pursuing a 'spectrum model' – which allows that certain personality and temperament features shape (fuzzily) the phenotypic picture of non-melancholic depression (see Fig. 3.2). For example, individuals who have an 'anxious worrying' personality style are more likely, when developing a non-melancholic depressive episode, to go quiet, to keep to themselves, and to have many prominent symptoms of anxiety, and thus, in terms of clinical features, show the classical picture of 'anxious depression'. Our spectrum model effectively argues that Axis II components (i.e. personality) influence Axis I phenomenology (i.e. symptoms), presumably because of shared psychobiological determinants. Such a model may assist the clinician; for example, a picture of anxious depression suggests that the patient may have an anxious worrying personality predisposing to depression. After assisting their depressive condition, the clinician may then consider whether there is anything that should be done to modulate that personality style to increase their resilience. Nevertheless, the model lacks the precision that is required to define clinical sub-sets at the primary level. Why? Firstly, because such 'symptom patterns' are intrinsically imprecise and diffuse. Secondly, because surface features are not always 'symptoms', sometimes alternately reflecting coping responses, homoeostatic mechanisms, and

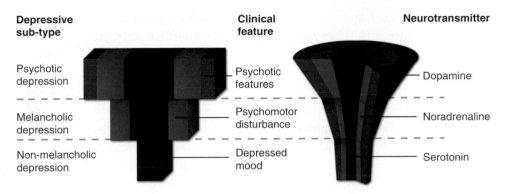

Fig. 3.3 Our structural and functional models of the three principal depressive sub-types.

other components, as we will later consider in relation to 'atypical depression'. Thus, we favour a primary 'bottom-up' model (weighted to aetiology) rather than a 'top-down' model (weighted to clinical features), in terms of greater explanatory power in modelling the non-melancholic disorders. As noted, we also consider the implications of a composite 'spectrum' model linking personality and clinical symptoms.

Our hierarchical model of the three principal depressive sub-types is primarily a 'structural' one, which, we suggest (Malhi et al., 2004) is likely to be underpinned and driven by differential 'functional' processes. We speculate (see Fig. 3.3) that there are likely to be differential neurotransmitter contributions to the three classes, with psychotic depression having a greater perturbation of dopaminergic function, melancholic depression of noradrenergic neurotransmitter function, and the non-melancholic disorders of serotonergic neurotransmitter dysfunction. This model might help to explain differential treatment gradients that we consider in subsequent chapters. Support for the model (albeit from an imprecise literature described in subsequent chapters) includes:

(i)   The non-differentiation of most treatments (antidepressant drug or other) for the non-melancholic class.

(ii) The greater efficacy of dual action and broad action antidepressants compared to selective serotonin reuptake inhibitors (SSRIs) for melancholic depression.

(iii) The fact that combination antipsychotic and antidepressant medication (i.e. broad action strategies) are far more effective than either alone for the management of psychotic depression.

The model therefore assumes the recruitment of differing proportions of key neurotransmitters to each of the three classes.

To the degree that psychotic and melancholic depression can be viewed as quintessentially biological and categorical disorders, and therefore conceptually simpler to diagnose and manage, we briefly consider some diagnostic and management recommendations for each in the following separate chapters.

Tackling the non-melancholic disorders is more problematic. Winokur (1991) suggested that a key objective of depression research should be to 'identify separate etiologies that in turn could translate into specific treatments'. While the aphorism that 'migraine is not due to an insufficiency of aspirin' reminds us that aetiology does not relate directly to treatment, some degree of linkage might be anticipated. Thus, we argue that it is of key importance to model the non-melancholic disorders according to their aetiological contribution, and we favour a model weighting three key interactive components: the individual's self-esteem, personality style, and triggering stressors. The model allows the development of a more rational approach to the management of those disorders that lie within the overall heterogeneous non-melancholic class. Each of these components to the model will be considered in separate chapters before moving to management nuances for non-melancholic depression. This is not to argue that personality, self-esteem, and triggering life event stressors are irrelevant to psychotic and melancholic depression, for we do accept that stressful events and personality may contribute to the onset and persistence of such conditions in some individuals. But, as we do not view them as primary aetiological drivers of those conditions, we detail their potential contributory role only in relation to the non-melancholic disorders, the focus of this book.

Sub-typing algorithm

1. Is the patient depressed? (Pursue depressed mood, self-criticism, and loss of self-esteem)
2. Does the patient have clinical depression? (Pursue severity and duration of symptoms, and impaired functioning)
3. Does the patient have psychotic depression? (Pursue psychotic features such as delusions, over-valued ideas of guilt, and feeling that he/she deserves to be punished. Is there severe of profound PMD, which may prevent psychotic features being elicited?)
4. Does the patient have melancholic depression? (In addition to a severely depressed mood, PMD should be evident)
5. Does the patient have a non-melancholic depression? (Psychotic features and PMD should not be able to be elicited. Should not have a bipolar history)

Part II

The diagnosis and management of melancholic and psychotic depression

Management of melancholic depression

Introduction

We view melancholic depression as a quintessential biological 'disease', and therefore preferentially responsive to biologically weighted treatments. As noted earlier, episodes may be precipitated or triggered by stressors such as interpersonal or work crises (and particularly those occurring early on in the life of the disorder), or may occur without any seeming trigger (i.e. 'endogenous' in the old terminology). For some individuals, there may be a seasonal predilection, with episodes being more likely to occur in spring, perhaps because of the rapid increase in luminosity stimulating the pineal gland. The point here is that 'stressors' may operate across a number of parameters.

For those with a lifetime unipolar course (episodes of melancholic depression only and no 'highs'), onset is rare at a young age, with episodes being more likely to commence in middle age or later. In those whose lifetime course is bipolar, episodes of melancholic or psychotic depression *can* occur at a much younger age, including in the teen years. We have a working principle (which, like most principles, is waiting rejection by a rush of exceptions) that: an episode of melancholic or psychotic depression in an individual aged less than 40 years of age is indicative of bipolar disorder being either present or being likely in the future. For such young subjects, we encourage close questioning about features of 'highs'. Further, numerous studies (see Parker & Hadzi-Pavlovic, 1996) have established that, when an individual with bipolar disorder develops depression, they have a very high probability of developing either a melancholic or psychotic depression, indicating a strong risk to the more biological expressions of depression. However, common sense indicates that those who have such a lifetime pattern of melancholic or psychotic depression, are, as for any other individual, also capable of developing non-melancholic episodes. For example, a woman with classical episodes of melancholic depression over the years presented on one occasion with a quite differing picture. Her husband had suddenly left her, and this had precipitated a reactive non-melancholic condition which the patient recognized as being distinctly different from previous episodes of depression.

In this chapter we define key clinical features of melancholia, offer a model for considering rational treatments and then focus on management strategies for unipolar melancholia.

Diagnosing melancholia

'Endogeneity symptoms' were held for a long time to be useful markers of melancholic depression. These included features such as early morning wakening, appetite and weight loss, and diurnal variation (i.e. mood and energy being worse in the morning). Regrettably, however, such symptoms have low specificity. As demonstrated in several of our studies (Parker & Hadzi-Pavlovic, 1996), while they may have a reasonably high prevalence in melancholic depression, their prevalence in the non-melancholic disorders may be similar or, if increased, only marginally so. Their utility is further compromised by self-report biases. Many patients with non-melancholic disorders will affirm endogeneity symptoms when questioned, either because of their non-specificity or because they wish to ensure that the clinician appreciates that they have a serious disorder, so that they therefore tend to acknowledge most features inquired about or rate their presence as more severe than might be judged objectively.

Symptoms of melancholic depression

Some symptoms strike us clinically as being more useful than others including:

(a) A categorically non-reactive mood or reporting only a superficial or transient response to potentially mood-lifting situations.

(b) Distinct anhedonia, or inability to expect or find pleasure in any putatively pleasurable event, although we have not found clear support for the suggestion that anticipatory anhedonia may be more specific to melancholia than consummatory anhedonia.

(c) Marked concentration impairment, with the individual finding it extremely difficult or impossible to attend to basic tasks like reading a book, and who often describe their brain as feeling very 'foggy'. In addition, they tend to experience profound anergia and physical inability to function, which can reach a state perceived to be like a 'mechanical failure'. In the past, terms such as 'paralysis of the will' were used to capture this key feature. Thus, individuals who are usually 'up and going' at

Fig. 4.1 Melancholic
depression.

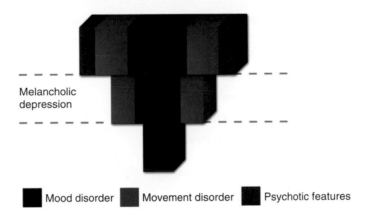

Melancholic
depression

■ Mood disorder   ■ Movement disorder   ■ Psychotic features

a reasonable hour and industrious across the day, may state that they find it extremely difficult to even get out of bed and to do basic things like showering.

While such symptoms have a moderate level of utility, regrettably they do not have high specificity, at least when we attempt to assess them as symptoms. We have previously argued (Parker & Hadzi-Pavlovic, 1996) that the key specific feature for the diagnosis of melancholia is observable psychomotor disturbance (PMD) (see Fig. 4.1).

We emphasise that PMD needs to be rated by an external observer rather than being assessed as a symptom as it is subject to self-report biases. Thus, if we ask depressed individuals (with melancholic or non-melancholic depression) whether they feel slowed down, most will affirm such symptoms (so that sub-typing specificity is potentially lost). The specificity of PMD is far more impressive, however, when rated behaviourally by observation. Our model is a 'trunk and branch' one (Fig. 4.2), with a central cognitive processing component (reflected by a lack of interactiveness and by evident impairment of attention and concentration). The motoric component is either retardation and/or agitation. Retardation is evidenced, for example, by slow speech, latency in responding to questions and in undertaking simple actions (such as getting out of a chair), poverty of speech, lack of facial reactivity (with patients generally losing the 'light in their eyes'), and clear non-reactivity to attempts to cheer the individual up. While 'agitation' is experienced symptomatically (with individuals feeling profoundly distressed and often describing epigastric churning and an inability to sit still) it is better viewed (and therefore measured) as the outward motor expression of their mental perturbation. Agitated individuals appear bewildered, perplexed, or puzzled. They tend to be preoccupied with issues that they see as extremely distressing but which, to the observer, appear to be relatively trivial. In addition to appearing apprehensive

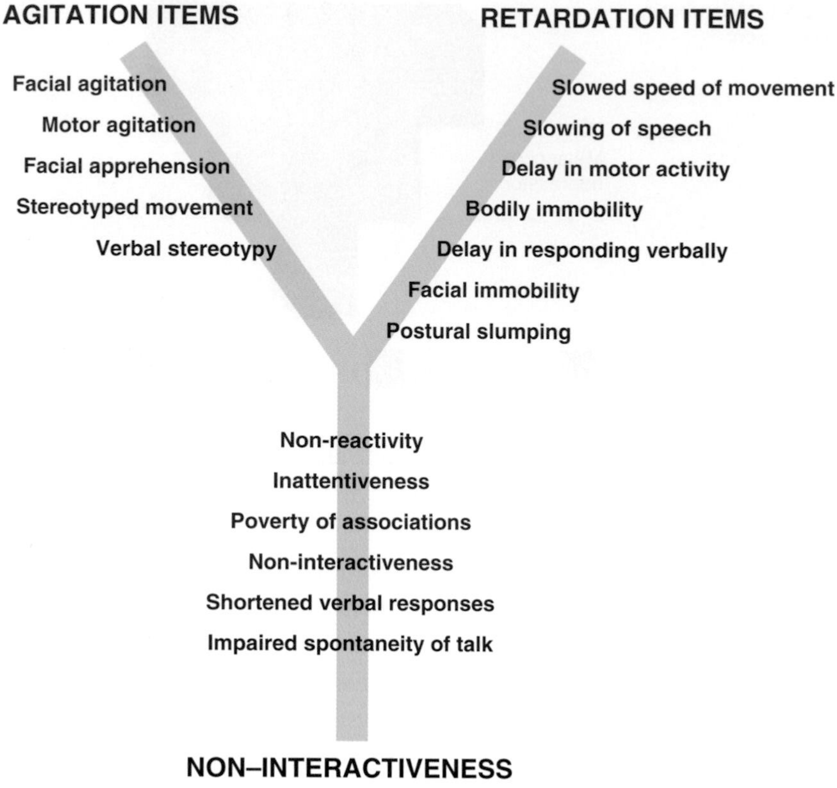

Fig. 4.2 The CORE
model of PMD.

AGITATION ITEMS

Facial agitation

Motor agitation

Facial apprehension

Stereotyped movement

Verbal stereotypy

RETARDATION ITEMS

Slowed speed of movement

Slowing of speech

Delay in motor activity

Bodily immobility

Delay in responding verbally

Facial immobility

Postural slumping

Non-reactivity

Inattentiveness

Poverty of associations

Non-interactiveness

Shortened verbal responses

Impaired spontaneity of talk

NON–INTERACTIVENESS

at times, they tend to show slow writhing movements (of hands and some-times of legs), and may be quite unable to sit or stay still, sometimes pacing up and down. Their talk has a characteristic coda, with morbidly repetitive or perseverative concerns, whereby they constantly seek, but appear generally inaccessible to reassurance. Importuning is common in severe expressions of melancholia (e.g. the individual repetitively asking 'What is going to become of me?'). Appendix 2 provides further information about the 'CORE' (measure of PMD signs) (Parker & Hadzi-Pavlovic, 1996) instructions and rating rules.

The CORE measure comprises a central 'non-interactiveness' and cogni-tive processing scale, and two arborising motoric scales assessing agitation and retardation.

Clinically, those with melancholic depression show one of two patterns:

(i) retardation only,

(ii) a base of retardation with superimposed epochs of agitation.

That subdivision (into retardation and agitation) does not appear, how-ever, to have many clinical implications, so that we use total CORE scores rather than sub-scale scores to determine melancholia. Certainly, those in the agitated sub-group are somewhat more likely to experience psychotic features at the worst of their episode. They also appear somewhat more likely to receive an incorrect diagnosis. Thus, we have seen many patients with agitated melancholia who have been misdiagnosed as having an anxiety state and who have been encouraged to have a course of relaxation therapy, transcendental mediation, or yoga – without benefit.

We have previously argued (Parker & Hadzi-Pavlovic, 1996) that observable PMD is both 'necessary and sufficient' for the diagnosis of melancholia: 'necessary' in that those with true melancholia always have a level of observable PMD and 'sufficient' in that PMD subsumes endogeneity symptoms (particularly those noted above) and effectively makes their contribution redundant. The latter is not entirely surprising, as a non-reactive mood, anhedonia and profound anergia would appear logical symptomatic expressions of PMD. However, since our early research studies were published, some caveats have emerged. While observable PMD was an extremely specific marker in those studies, most of our samples involved middle aged and elderly people. We now have the view that younger patients with true melancholia may not show observable PMD to such a clear degree, particularly those who have a unipolar course. Most, however, will describe the subjective concomitants of PMD, such as distinct impairment in concentration, anergia, and 'mechanical failure', as well as anhedonia and a non-reactive mood. If this age effect is a valid interpretation, it could reflect the phenotypic picture of melancholia changing with age (i.e. observable PMD becoming more distinct and severe), possibly reflecting progressive recruitment of monoaminergic systems with age. We shall return to this issue shortly, as we believe that there are major implications for management.

Functional and structural melancholia

We have also argued (Parker & Hadzi-Pavlovic, 1996) for two differing (but not necessarily mutually exclusive) trajectories to the development of 'melancholia', one weighting a functional aetiology and the other a 'structural' component. In those with 'functional melancholia' (Fig. 4.3) there is often a family history of a biological mood disorder. They tend to have their first episode at a younger age (i.e. before the age of 60 years), brain scans such as magnetic resonance imaging (MRI) are unlikely to identify any structural lesion, and, when commenced on an appropriate antidepressant or having electroconvulsive therapy (ECT) initiated, they tend to respond fairly smoothly and have high response rates to such interventions. By contrast, those with 'structural melancholia' (Fig. 4.4) tend to have their first episode at a much older age (i.e. 60–80 years), and be more likely to have a family

Fig. 4.3 Functional melancholia (i.e. normal brain scan).

Increased family history of affective disorder; MRI usually shows no abnormality, and patients generally have a smooth response to physical treatments

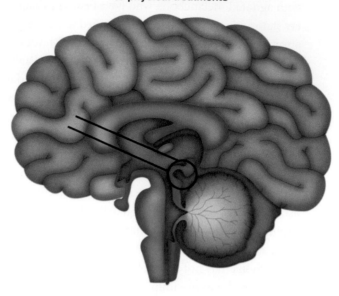

Fig. 4.4 Structural melancholia (i.e. evidence of hyperintensities and/or reduction in basal ganglia volume).

Usually older at first onset, increased chance of a cerebrovascular and cardiovascular family history; ApoE risk factor more relevant; MRI likely to identify hyperintensities and decreased basal ganglia volume. Standard doses of antidepressants and frequencies of ECT may induce delirium

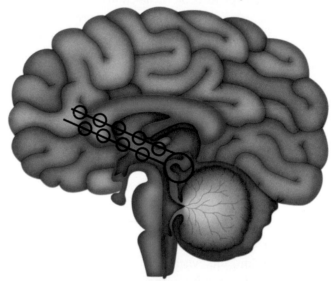

history of cerebrovascular or cardiovascular problems, ApoE allele abnormalities and, on structural brain scanning, evidence of white matter hyperintensities (indicative of microvascular changes), and somewhat more likely to have a reduction in basal ganglia volume (particularly of the caudate and putamen). They may respond well initially to a physical treatment (i.e. anti-depressant drugs or ECT) but, following any such remission, episodes tend to become more frequent while their response to intervention is progressively diminished. Here, our model assumes that the 'melancholia' is an early marker of a presaging dementia in this sub-set.

As detailed previously (Parker & Hadzi-Pavlovic, 1996), such a model for 'melancholia' assumes that certain neural circuits linking the basal ganglia with the prefrontal cortex are, when interrupted (functionally and/or struc-turally), likely to result in a triad of clinical features (i.e. depression, concen-tration impairment, and motoric expressions of PMD). If the disruption is essentially functionally derived, presumed perturbations in relevant neuro-transmitters might then be assumed to underpin the disrupted circuit and to be likely to normalise in response to appropriate physical treatments (e.g. certain antidepressant drugs and ECT). If there is an additional structural component, whether reflecting an early dementia or not, the capacity of redressing the structural abnormality by antidepressant drugs or ECT is clearly limited, thus explaining the generally worse trajectory (e.g. drug and ECT-induced delirium in a percentage) and overall worse prognosis for those with 'structural melancholia'.

Acute management of unipolar melancholic depression

As noted, we prioritise a biologically weighted approach to the management of melancholia. This is supported by response rates of 60–80% for physical treat-ments such as ECT and antidepressant drugs in clinical effectiveness studies as against a placebo/spontaneous remission rate of some 10%, a striking gradi-ent. The literature base for quantifying the efficacy of the psychotherapies is problematic (largely reflecting the variable definition of 'melancholia') but we would suggest that they have no primary role, and more over, they contribute, in combination with a physical treatment, to a 'good clinical care' model, although augmentation capacities would also need to be conceded.

While it is commonly suggested that all antidepressants are of equal effi-cacy for managing 'depression', we believe that there is increasing evidence challenging that view, as considered in earlier chapters. If the differing anti-depressant classes do differ in terms of their antidepressant effectiveness, we suggest that this is far more likely to operate across the 'more biological disorders' (including melancholic depression) than hold for the non-melancholic disorders. Other observers (American Psychiatric Association, 2000) have suggested that broader-spectrum antidepressants (such as tricyclic antidepressants, TCA) are more effective in those with 'more severe' depres-sion and for hospital inpatients. We see those two features as indirect proxies

Table 4.1 Suggested model for managing acute unipolar melancholia.

If no previous medication
- **Step I**: SSRI if 'young' and no distinct PMD. Dual-action antidepressant if older and/or distinct PMD
- **Step II**: Dual-action drug if SSRI trialled and failed
- **Step III**: TCA or MAOI if dual action drug trialled and failed
- **Step IV**: ECT (other reasons may advance its case)

If previous antidepressants failed?
- Try one other drug in that class or move to next untested step

Augmentation
- Low-dose Olanzapine (i.e. 2.5–5 mg) after Steps I, II, or III (If it is to work, expect improvement in 1–7 days, otherwise cease. If seeming to drive improvement, particularly in inducing a rapid response, try to cease after 1 week of remission)
- Lithium or thyroid hormone (if Step III fails)

of the greater likelihood of the melancholic sub-type and that, overall, broader-spectrum antidepressants are more likely to have a higher response rate than narrow-action antidepressants. Such data provide indirect support for our 'functional model' (noted earlier) which imputes a distinct noradrenergic (in addition to serotonergic) contribution. Nevertheless, this does not of necessity argue for always initiating treatment for melancholia with a broad-action antidepressant.

Our sequencing model is illustrated in Table 4.1. The first step allows that the patient might initially receive:

(i)   a narrow-action antidepressant (such as a selective serotonin reuptake inhibitor, SSRI), particularly for those patients with 'functional melancholia' and younger patients whose PMD is not too severe;

(ii) a dual-action antidepressant.

If this strategy is successful, we would anticipate evidence of some improvement by 2 weeks. If, by contrast, the patient has previously received a narrow-action antidepressant such as an SSRI and shown a poor response and/or has severe PMD, there is an argument for commencing with a dual-action or even broader-action antidepressant at Step 1. If monotherapy is to be pursued, the model recommends that, if the dual-action antidepressant fails to effect any improvement after 2–3 weeks, a TCA or a monoamine oxidase inhibitor (MAOI) should be considered. If these strategies fail, then ECT should be considered. Clearly, ECT might need to be considered at an earlier stage, particularly if the individual has previously shown a good response to it, is in a parlous physical state (e.g. dehydrated from lack of fluid intake), experiencing profound mental distress (e.g. extreme agitation), or for other logical clinical reasons.

Augmentation strategies (such as adding lithium or a thyroid hormone to the antidepressant) are generally considered and implemented after two or three antidepressant classes have been trialled without success. While potentially useful, their success rate in our hands is not particularly high (being in the order of 10% or less). We have had considerably greater success (Parker, 2001; Parker & Malhi, 2001; Parker et al., 2005) in augmenting with atypical antipsychotic drugs where, for those with melancholic depression, the success rate of such augmentation is more in the order of 30–40%. We suspect that the differing antipsychotic drugs differ in their capacity to augment antidepressants and that there are some important nuances to their prescription that would benefit from more applied research.

Examples can be provided from our considerable experience with Olanzapine. Here we find two patterns of 'successful augmentation'. Firstly, a sub-set of individuals with melancholia who, when receiving an antidepressant that is 'potentially' therapeutic (accepting that response is difficult to predict *a priori* at the individual level), respond to low-dose Olanzapine (i.e. 2.5–5 mg) at somewhere between 1 and 7 days after initiation (i.e. a delayed response is unusual). The relevance of referring to a 'potentially therapeutic' antidepressant is as follows. We have had some patients, who have shown no response to augmentation when on a narrow-action antidepressant SSRI, or even to augmentation by a dual-action drug but, when placed on a broader-action antidepressant such as a TCA or MAOI, have shown a very rapid response to such augmentation. Thus, we do not assume that a lack of response to a narrow-action antidepressant necessitates a lack of potential to respond to broader-action ones. If complete remission occurs, we cease the Olanzapine within a few days and then seek to determine whether the remission is sustained while maintaining the antidepressant at the same dose or (subsequently) at a lower dose. Sometimes, such remission is not maintained and there are advantages to considering whether the antidepressant dose should be increased (with or without repeat augmentation). On occasions, successful and rapid low-dose augmentation with an atypical antipsychotic can precipitate a minor (and generally transient) 'high'. Such 'switching' is commonly missed as both the patient and the clinician are focused on 'remission'. When a patient reports 'It's a miracle, I haven't felt so good for a long time', a clinician might (not unreasonably) feel a profound sense of relief and not pursue 'switching'. As noted, this is generally not a substantive issue, but can argue for continuing the augmentation, at least until the 'high' has settled.

Secondly, there is another sub-set of patients who obtain partial remission status with an atypical antipsychotic augmenting drug, but who generally require a much higher dose (i.e. 10–20 mg Olanzapine) or another atypical antipsychotic drug to achieve that state, and who tend to relapse when it is tapered or ceased.

If augmentation of a narrow-action (i.e. SSRI) or dual-action drug with an atypical antipsychotic fails, as noted, we may cease that antidepressant, and trial a broader-action TCA or MAOI for a few days to 2 weeks and, if no evidence of any improvement, again augment that drug with an atypical antipsychotic drug. In a recent study (Parker et al., 2005) where we examined whether there was any responsivity or speed of action advantage to the co-prescription of Olanzapine and an antidepressant (as against prescribing an antidepressant alone), we did find that the later addition of Olanzapine to antidepressant non-responders was associated with rapid remission. This raised the question as to whether augmentation with an atypical antipsychotic might achieve greater benefit when the antidepressant is already 'on board', as was described in the early studies of lithium augmentation.

Maintenance issues for unipolar melancholic depression

Upon recovery, maintenance medication is generally required for extended periods to reduce the chance of relapse. While the management priority focuses on the use of biologically weighted treatments (such as antidepressant drugs and ECT), we clearly accept the importance of considering a whole range of other issues and approaches early in management. These include considering the need to hospitalise the patient, need to provide appropriate reassurance and a positive prognosis to the patient and their relatives, need for vigilance to ensure the patient's safety, and appropriate counselling about how to deal with current stresses such as inability to get to work or to relate to family members. Once the acute episode has remitted, a whole range of contributory factors – as well as consequences of the mood state – may well benefit from attention, and it is at this stage that pluralistic management comes into its own as the bedrock for progress. While we do not see any primary contribution from personality style in 'causing' the disorder, the patient's personality may impact on their adherence to treatment, on the day-to-day management and perhaps even in response to differing medications. For example, perfectionistic patients may, after some improvement, start wrestling again with the triggers that had preoccupied them and contributed to depression onset, and effectively drive themselves back into a full episode. Such nuances of personality style are considered later in this book.

The additional contribution of less orthodox treatment components is problematic, preventing any clear recommendations. Two examples: depressed individuals are commonly encouraged to exercise and to 'keep busy'. We have seen patients with melancholic depression who have obtained distinct benefit from a structured exercise program, in that getting out of bed and walking around the block has helped to distract them to some degree from their pervading thoughts. Again, for those who have shown a distinct but not complete remission, and who may have some residual diurnal variation of mood and energy, exercise on getting out of bed may over-ride those residual symptoms with benefit. We have also seen others who have found such strategies to be counter-productive and where it has appeared preferable (for all concerned) to allow the individual to lie in bed and wait until the treatment had worked its benefits. Secondly, we have had patients with agitated melancholia who, in addition to reporting benefit from medication for their agitation, have reported additional or even superior benefit from relaxation training. Prescriptive rules for management, and even broad recommendations, are therefore problematic in relation to non-physical treatments. Clinical care is generally then a mix of relatively obligatory components (e.g. medication, regular review) and those facultative components that are negotiated with the patients and established, often on a trial and error basis, as beneficial to that individual.

5

Management of psychotic depression

Classification

The nosological status of psychotic depression is unclear. If its definition is determined by a unique specifier (i.e. psychotic features) this argues for a categorical sub-type. In the past, however, such a diagnosis tended to be applied, particularly in the UK, to patients with 'severe' depressive conditions, and did not necessarily require psychotic features. Similarly, in the USA, Minter and Mandel (1979) suggested that psychotic depression had 'Come to mean the same as "endogenous depression" or to mean a severe depression, usually with endogenous symptomatology, not necessarily with symptoms of psychosis'. Viewing 'psychotic depression' as synonymous with 'melancholia' suggests, in essence, that both were viewed as 'more severe' expressions of depression and that the presence or absence of psychotic features was not seen as being of great clinical relevance. We suggest that, phenomenologically, most of the clinical features observed in psychotic depression are ones observed in those with melancholia (albeit generally more severe), apart from psychotic features, and this could argue for the condition being a sub-set of a broader melancholic class. However, in addition, and as noted shortly, psychotic depression is distinctly less likely than melancholia to respond to an antidepressant alone. This characteristic, together with the class specifier (psychotic symptoms) provides the argument for class status.

Clinical diagnosis

Psychotic features are mandatory for the diagnosis (see Fig. 5.1) but, as many patients with the condition have profound psychomotor disturbance (PMD) (sometimes to the extent of being mute and catatonic), the presence of such features may not be volunteered or readily identified.

Fig. 5.1 Psychotic
depression.

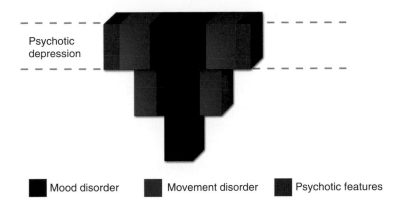

Psychotic
depression

■ Mood disorder   ■ Movement disorder   ■ Psychotic features

Interviewing family members or other corroborative witnesses may assist, while interviewing such patients following improvement may then establish that such features were present at episode nadir. Thus, when PMD is profound, suspect psychotic depression and consider managing accordingly.

Delusions are more common psychotic features than hallucinations, while over-valued ideas are frequent. Patients, who merely have over-valued ideas, rather than frank delusions and hallucinations, are particularly problematic in allowing a confident diagnosis, as deciding whether an over-valued idea as against a depressive rumination exists is neither theoretically nor practically straightforward. Guilt is the commonest theme underlying over-valued ideas and delusions, and can be the most useful conduit for questioning. Patients who have not thought about a possible indiscretion or incident for decades (e.g. cheating on their income tax, having a termination of pregnancy) may ruminate with profound guilt and with little relief from such thoughts, and with many considering dire action. We have had patients attempt suicide, or turn up at police stations and perturb their family by stating that they deserve punishment for objectively minor indiscretions that are viewed by the patient as evil acts. Thus, in patients where psychotic features are either denied or not volunteered, pursuit of the diagnostic possibility is often best assisted by questioning whether the individual feels 'guilty' or feels either that they 'deserve to be punished' or 'are being punished'.

Nihilistic and somatic delusions are also common. For example, somatic features may involve a mistaken belief involving cancer, or that their 'bowels have turned to cement'. Hallucinations may be compatible with the delusional thinking, with the individual hearing voices stating that they are evil or worthless. Psychotic features can also be at variance from the depressive theme (e.g. the individual might be convinced that people are watching them, or that gas is being pumped under the floorboards of their home). In our review (Parker & Hadzi-Pavlovic, 1996) of numerous studies examining the phenomenology of psychotic depression, we found that mood-incongruent psychotic features were slightly more likely than mood-congruent ones. Thus, there is a risk that some individuals with psychotic depression may be diagnosed as having schizophrenia (or dementia). The longitudinal course, together with symptom-free intervals, is a useful distinguishing marker of the diagnosis.

PMD is evident and, almost invariably, more severe, than in melancholic depression without psychotic features. Severe cognitive functioning limitations can suggest a dementia. While this may commonly be a form of 'pseudo-dementia', late onset and other features may suggest the likelihood of 'structural melancholia', and presage a 'true' dementia.

An agitated picture is slightly more common than a retarded picture in those with psychotic depression, and with importuning ('What is going to become of me?') a frequent manifestation. Preoccupations about past indiscretions, incipient penury, and about quite banal topics (e.g. 'How can I afford to have a haircut?') are common. While not of major differentiating importance, constipation is not an uncommon symptom, even prior to prescription of any medication that might have such a side effect. We suspect that, just as such patients have profound PMD affecting general motoric functioning, PMD can also affect gastrointestinal motility, and so result in constipation. Such a symptom can then serve as a nidus for developing a preoccupation that there has to be a malignant reason for the constipation, and so possibly explain many patients' convictions about their bowels having turned to cement or becoming cancerous. Interestingly, relieving the constipation in such patients can cause a temporary improvement in their mood state and preoccupations.

While those with melancholia appear somewhat more likely to show diurnal variation of mood and energy, with both being worse in the morning and improving as the day goes on, such a feature is less common in psychotic depression. As individuals with this condition enter an episode, they may show diurnal variation but, as the disorder becomes more severe, their mood and energy levels tend to persist without variation across the day, and with diurnal variation only returning to the melancholic pattern of early morning worsening when there has been some improvement in the condition.

We have long had the clinical impression that those who develop psychotic depression are more likely to have an obsessional, perfectionistic, and anxious worrying personality style, but in formal studies we have failed to confirm such personality differences. Any over-represented predisposing personality styles remain to be established.

Table 5.1 Suggested model for managing psychotic depression.

- **Step I**: Antidepressant + antipsychotic drug
- **Step II**: ECT (other reasons may advance its case as a Step I strategy)

Acute management of unipolar psychotic depression

As for melancholia, the management priority is to biologically weighted treatments; that is, psychotropic drugs and/or electroconvulsive therapy (ECT) (see Table 5.1). There have been two meta-analyses (Spiker et al., 1985; Parker et al., 1992) that have quantified quite similar gradients across differing treatments. Prescription of an antidepressant drug alone was associated with improvement in about one-quarter of subjects, an antipsychotic alone of 30%, as against 80% for their combination. The combination benefit provides indirect support for our 'functional model' which imputes, for psychotic depression, a greater dopaminergic and noradrenergic contribution, rather than a dominant and specific serotonergic contribution. ECT had a similar 80% response as for combination antidepressant and antipsychotic, although there was the suggestion that bilateral ECT was slightly more powerful than unilateral ECT. As those studies are somewhat dated, most of the analyses would have been based on tricyclic antidepressants (TCA), monoamine oxidase inhibitor (MAOI) antidepressants and the typical antipsychotic drugs. As yet, there are no meta-analyses considering whether the atypical antipsychotic drugs have any differential responsiveness compared to the typicals, and similarly, no clear-cut database exists for the newer antidepressants. We suspect, however, that narrow-action antidepressants would be less effective than TCAs and MAOIs.

Several studies have established that this condition has a very low spontaneous or placebo response rate (in the order of 5%), while the chance of misadventure and suicide is high, arguing commonly for hospitalisation. Other management strategies, and the need to segment and sequence differing treatment modalities, have been covered in the previous section dealing with the acute management of melancholia.

Maintenance issues for unipolar psychotic depression

In our clinical management, we usually maintain both the antipsychotic and antidepressant medications until the patient has been well for about a month, then we cautiously attempt to withdraw the antipsychotic drug, which, if maintained at the level required during the depressive episode, may by then be causing excessive sedation. As the psychotic features tend to show a remarkable consistency across episodes, any individual patient's sentinel preoccupation (e.g. 'I am an evil person for cheating on my income tax') can often serve as a review marker to determine whether the individual is generally well, has residual disorder, or has an incipient or developing recurrence.

Whilst first-line treatments for psychotic melancholia are necessarily biologically weighted, social and psychological interventions may still play a crucial role in the recovery process. The involvement of family members in ensuring safety, rehabilitation, and in assisting treatment compliance can help to allay anxiety and facilitate specific intervention strategies, such as keeping regular appointments with the treating physician, especially in the early phases of recovery.

6

Bipolar melancholic or psychotic depression

While the recommendations given in Chapters 4 and 5 have been predicated on unipolar patterns, the management of those who have a bipolar lifetime course of melancholic or psychotic depression is much more complicated. As noted earlier, those with bipolar disorder are highly likely (approximately 80%) to have melancholic or psychotic depression patterns when depressed. More specifically, bipolar II patients tend to have melancholic depression, but not psychotic depression; while up to 50% of those with bipolar I disorder will experience psychotic depression. The distinctions between differing bipolar disorders make management even more complicated.

Firstly, distinctions between the disorders may not be dimensional (i.e. bipolar II being viewed as a 'less severe' disorder than bipolar I) as generally assumed. A recent review (Hadjipavlou et al., 2004) indicated that, while the 'highs' may not be distinctly disturbing in bipolar II disorder, both the course and the depressive episodes may be just as 'severe' for the I and II expressions, while those with bipolar II may have longer episodes and lengthier periods of sub-syndromal dysfunction, as well as be at greater risk of suicide.

Secondly, those authors concluded that basing treatment recommendations for those with bipolar II on bipolar I studies 'may prove to be at the very least hasty and premature, if not inappropriate'. Thirdly, while it is difficult enough to interpret randomised controlled trials (RCTs) for the management of unipolar depression, the situation is predictably more complicated for bipolar disorder, when patients may present when 'high', when depressed (and with differing depressive conditions) and when in mixed states, providing permutations and combinations that constrain empirically derived guidelines.

Fourthly, while most studies collect data at intervals (whether weekly or even longer), people with bipolar disorder are commonly oscillating at high frequency, so that we lack useful strategies for assessing such oscillating mood states over brief periods of time. Fifthly, the management of bipolar disorder requires a frame of reference lasting months and usually years, particularly when episodes may only occur every few months, or longer, so that examining the impact of any medication and medication change becomes problematic. Sixthly, we suggest that the introduction of many new physical treatment approaches (e.g. atypical antipsychotic drugs, omega 3 fatty acids) for bipolar disorder are invoking new paradigms for conceptualisation and management considerations (i.e. do the atypical antipsychotic drugs act as mood stabilisers or via some other mechanism?). Finally, drug treatment (whether valid or not) is moving away from the rule of parsimony, with the management of bipolar disorder often involving the use of multiple medications, often of quite varying classes. As a consequence, our capacity to derive clear-cut management guidelines is limited.

As this book focuses more on non-melancholic disorders and on non-drug approaches, we do not consider psychopharmacological nuances for bipolar disorder (and bipolar melancholic or psychotic depression) in any detail. There are many excellent treatment guidelines that provide such information, for example the *2003 Consensus Guidelines* developed by the British Association for Psychopharmacology (BAP) (Goodwin et al., 2003), the STEP Program led by Gary Sachs (Sachs et al., 2000), and *Australasian Guidelines*, generated by Philip Mitchell (Mitchell et al., 2004).

However, we do offer some comments on issues that strike us as relevant to this subgroup. Firstly, bipolar disorder is far more common than is generally viewed, so that all depressed patients should be screened to determine whether their depressive illness has a unipolar or bipolar course and, if the latter, whether it shows a bipolar I or II pattern. Lack of identification more commonly reflects failure to ask probe questions rather than misdiagnosing true bipolar disorder as not present (e.g. for failing to have episodes of sufficient duration) or as some other condition (e.g. anxiety disorder, or an attention deficit disorder) or as merely reflecting a cyclothymic personality style. Our web site (blackdoginstitute.org.au) has a screening questionnaire that can be used by clinicians or by consumers to assist clarifying the probability.

Secondly, and as noted earlier, for those who have bipolar disorder, 80% of the characteristically depressive episodes are psychotic or melancholic depression. Thirdly, in addition to determining what antidepressant might be warranted, there is commonly the need to consider antidepressant augmentation strategies (which range from pharmacological ones such as mood stabilisers through to cognitive behavioural and psychoeducational 'stay well' programs, with each having been shown to have distinct benefits to long-term management). For choice of possible mood stabiliser (e.g. lamotrigine being more effective for predominating depressive than manic episodes; atypical antipsychotic drugs having the converse profile), we again refer to the *BAP Guidelines* (Goodwin et al., 2003).

With regard to those who are acutely depressed, many treatment guidelines are extremely cautious about the use of antidepressants, being concerned about the capacity of the antidepressant to cause a manic 'switch', once regarded clinically as the *sine qua non* of an effective antidepressant. Many recommendations argue against any use of an antidepressant until a mood stabiliser has been prescribed and until that drug has achieved a therapeutic level. A review of the literature (Parker & Parker, 2003) suggests to us, however, that the narrow-action (e.g. selective serotonin reuptake inhibitor, SSRI) and dual-action (e.g. serotonin-norepinephrine reuptake inhibitor, SNRI) antidepressant drugs are far less likely to have such a side effect than the broader tricyclic antidepressants (TCA) and monoamine oxidase inhibitor (MAOI) drugs. Thus, focussing now on bipolar melancholic depression, we would treat the depressive episode akin to our treatment of a biological depressive disorder in those with a unipolar course (other than recognising the greater risk of TCAs and MAOIs inducing a manic 'switch') and not necessarily hold off introducing an antidepressant until a mood stabiliser had been established. If an antidepressant alone did not induce remission we would add an atypical antipsychotic drug after a brief interval to seek augmentation benefits and, if remission occurred, trial tapering and ceasing the latter after several weeks of euthymia (see Table 6.1). Electroconvulsive therapy (ECT) certainly needs to be considered in a small percentage of patients.

In terms of preventing melancholic depressive episodes in those with bipolar disorder, clinicians commonly work to the rule of parsimony, striving to use one mood stabiliser alone. Clinical experience and some recent studies suggest that many patients require and benefit from an ongoing antidepressant as well as one or more mood stabilisers, while the use of the atypical antipsychotic drugs as maintenance strategies (alone or in combination) is being increasingly examined. Thus, the management of those who experience bipolar depression is commonly complex and, as emphasised earlier, not readily reducible to straightforward procedures or guidelines. Clinicians dealing with such patients need to be aware that they are in for 'the long haul' in managing such patients, and while results may formally be less satisfactory than dealing with unipolar depressive disorders, such patients are extremely appreciative of close and thoughtful clinical attention.

Table 6.1 Suggested model for managing bipolar melancholic or psychotic depression.

- **Step I**: Initiate antidepressant strategies detailed for managing unipolar melancholic or psychotic depression but favour SSRI and dual-action antidepressants (due to risk of inducing switching with TCAs and MAOIs)
- **Step II**: Initiate mood stabilising strategies
- **Step III**: Once the patient is stabilised, review all medication in terms of dose and need for ongoing maintenance. Aim for use of mood stabilisers alone, or mood stabilisers plus an antidepressant or, if experiencing psychotic episodes of depression and mania, consider use of a low-dose atypical neuroleptic

Part III

An introduction to non-melancholic depression

7

Our model of non-melancholic depression

Unlike the psychotic and melancholic depressive disorders (which are characterised by distinct patterns of clinical features), the non-melancholic depressive disorders lack any specific depressive features, reflecting their class status as comprising a heterogeneous set of conditions sharing one obligatory feature (a depressed mood), and with their variegated expression reflecting the impact of life event stress on the individual's personality and self-esteem, and consequential coping repertoires (see Fig. 7.1).

Our model assumes less of a primacy of biological perturbations in the non-melancholic disorders than for melancholic and psychotic depression. We are not arguing, however, that the non-melancholic disorders are non-biological disorders – certain biological factors *may* contribute to the onset, while the consequential mood state and many of its correlates (e.g. anxiety) must have some biological underpinnings. Our emphasis is, however, on the key contributing factors.

In developing a model, we first detail a neurotransmitter model that is commonly used to explicate the biological substrate to depressive disorders. This will allow us to describe an analogous model for the development of non-melancholic depression, where self-esteem, a key construct of dysphoric

Fig. 7.1 Non-melancholic depression.

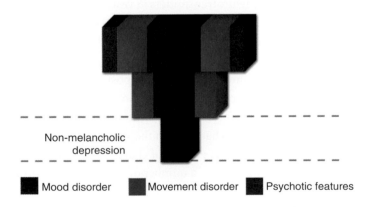

Non-melancholic depression

■ Mood disorder   ■ Movement disorder   ■ Psychotic features

mood, is 'switched off' when life event stressors are registered and processed, and interact with the individual's personality to result in a depressed state. Here, 'self-esteem expression' is modelled as being analogous to the biological concept of 'gene expression'; that is, the end stage of a process leading to self-esteem being decreased or maintained. Our psychotransmitter model specifies mechanistic processes linking stressful stimuli and differing personality styles as causes of non-melancholic depression, and so allows intervention points to be specified more rationally for salient treatment approaches.

It is important to bear in mind that this is a 'model' and, is, to a degree, metaphorical. While some of its components may be somewhat 'strained', it allows nuances of the non-melancholic disorders to be considered in some depth, and in relation to each other. The next section provides a brief reminder of the basic concepts of neurotransmitter activity to set the stage for a 'psychotransmitter model'.

Elements of neurotransmission

Chemical neurotransmission in the brain is responsible for regulating the expression of genes contained in neurons. These chemical processes are mediated by the movement of neurotransmitter molecules across the synaptic cleft separating the pre-synaptic neuron from the post-synaptic neuron. When neurotransmitter molecules reach the receiving neuron they cause a cascade of chemical reactions that ultimately result in genes located deep within the nucleus of the second neuron either being 'switched on' or 'switched off' (see Fig. 7.2). Gene expression can affect the working of the entire neuron, and its ability to communicate and interact with other neurons in the brain. Thus, gene expression is the fundamental end point.

In models of chemical neurotransmission, axons in a pre-synaptic neuron store neurotransmitters in vesicles located at their extremities. When stimulated by an electrical 'impulse', these vesicles discharge their contents (i.e. neurotransmitters) into the extra-cellular space between neurons. Once discharged into the extra-cellular space (or synaptic cleft), the neurotransmitters bombard receptors on the post-synaptic neuron and thus initiate a complex series of chemical reactions within the receiving neuron. Neurotransmitter 'receptor-binding', among other things, results in the opening or closing of 'ion channels' on the surface of the post-synaptic neuron. Ion channels control the passage of charged molecules to and from the neuron, which, in turn, initiate a number of other chemical processes within the cell (see Fig. 7.3).

Fig. 7.2 The neuro-
transmitter model.

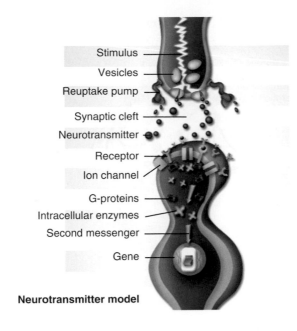

Stimulus
Vesicles
Reuptake pump
Synaptic cleft
Neurotransmitter
Receptor
Ion channel
G-proteins
Intracellular enzymes
Second messenger
Gene

Neurotransmitter model

Fig. 7.3 Receptor-
binding.

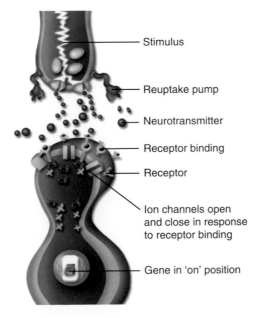

Stimulus

Reuptake pump

Neurotransmitter

Receptor binding

Receptor

Ion channels open
and close in response
to receptor binding

Gene in 'on' position

Within the synaptic cleft, neurotransmitter molecules that have not bound to receptors in the second neuron are re-absorbed by the pre-synaptic neuron through a 'reuptake pump' or destroyed by enzymes located in the synaptic cleft (see Fig. 7.4). Neurotransmitter molecules that are re-absorbed may also be destroyed by intracellular enzymes or re-packaged into vesicles for re-use.

Fig. 7.4 Neurotransmitter reuptake.

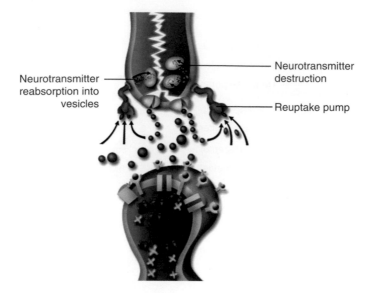

Fig. 7.5 Production of second messengers.

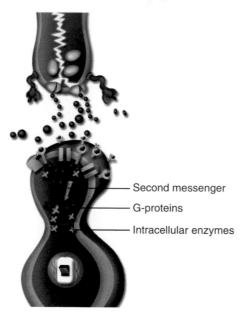

Neurotransmitters that have docked onto receptors are usually rapidly released so that they do not continue to stimulate the post-synaptic neuron.

Neurotransmitter molecules (or 'first messengers') that find their way to receptors on the post-synaptic neuron form a neurotransmitter-receptor complex which initiates a cascade of chemical reactions and involves other substances such as proteins (G-proteins) and intracellular enzymes. These chemical processes result in the production of another type of molecule referred to as a 'second messenger' (see Fig. 7.5). In some chemical reactions,

Fig. 7.6 Switching on the gene.

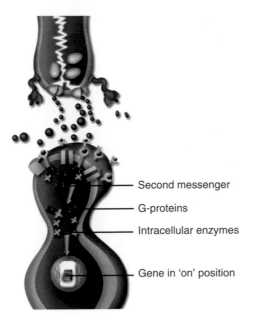

Second messenger

G-proteins

Intracellular enzymes

Gene in 'on' position

there can also be a third and fourth messenger. The second messenger together with a number of enzymes and other substances referred to as 'transcription factors' can also open and close ion channels. However, their primary function is to communicate with the DNA located in the nucleus to either 'switch on' or 'switch off' specific genes (see Fig. 7.6).

Activation of the post-synaptic neuron is dependent on a number of factors including the numbers of receptors on the cell membrane and whether the neurotransmitter being received acts as an 'agonist' (stimulating activity), 'partial agonist' (stimulating some activity such as partially opening ion channels) or 'antagonist' (blocking the effects of an agonist). If the post-synaptic neuron becomes over-stimulated, its response is to slow down the synthesis and transport of new receptors to the cell membrane and remove existing receptors from their sites of action. This process is referred to as 'down-regulation' and serves to attenuate the sequence of chemical reactions and lessens the likelihood of gene activation (see Fig. 7.7).

If, on the other hand, the post-synaptic neuron is under-stimulated, then it begins to synthesise and transport increased numbers of receptors to the cell membrane, thus effectively increasing the numbers and frequency of neurotransmitter 'hits'. This process, referred to as 'up-regulation' increases the pace of cellular activity and the likelihood of gene activation (see Fig. 7.8).

Neuronal activity may also be modulated by increasing or decreasing the density of dendritic branches. The natural 'pruning' of dendritic branches by specialised enzymes occurs when there are chronically low levels of neuronal

Fig. 7.7
Down-regulation.

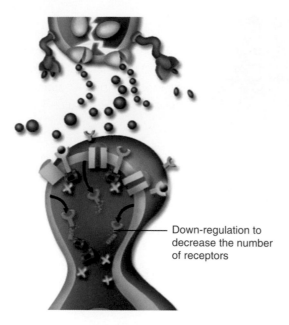

Down-regulation to
decrease the number
of receptors

Fig. 7.8
Up-regulation.

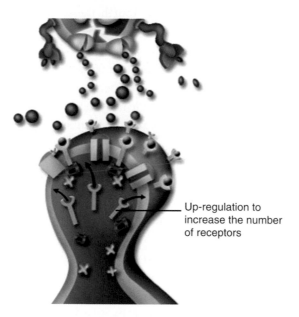

Up-regulation to
increase the number
of receptors

stimulation in the surrounding area. Additional branching occurs when there is a relatively high level of stimulation over a period of time. The main point from this overview is to indicate that neuronal transmission is extremely plastic, and can be modulated at both the intra- or extracellular levels.

Faulty neurotransmission: multiple components

As overviewed, the process of neuronal communication is extremely complex and there are multiple ways by which neurotransmission can be perturbed. Research has identified the most common problem areas to occur either at receptor sites or at the point of intracellular enzyme activity. Some of the common ways in which neuronal activity may be disrupted include the following:

1. Too much stimulation, for example, via ion channels which are inappropriately open, or if there are too many receptors, resulting in 'excitotoxicity', which can significantly disrupt cellular functioning or kill the neuron;
2. Malfunction at the receptor level, which can result in lack of binding of the neurotransmitter, and subsequent destruction of the neurotransmitter at the synapse;
3. An imbalance of several neurotransmitters competing for the same receptor complex;
4. Faulty connections from one neuron to the next so that effective communication between neurons is lost;
5. The natural pruning process of dendrites may go wrong so that neurons shrivel and ultimately die from lack of stimulation; or external agents (such as recreational drugs, caffeine or toxins that cross the blood-brain barrier) may affect the process of neurotransmission at the intra- and extracellular levels.

A 'psychotransmitter' model for non-melancholic depression

We can transpose elements of that chemical neurotransmitter model to consider 'causes' of non-melancholic depression, identifying analogous components as listed in Table 7.1 and illustrated in Fig. 7.9. Our psychotransmitter model uses the analogy of the neurotransmitter system to help explain how an individual's self-esteem acts as a barometer of mood state. In this context, self-esteem has both trait and state status. If self-esteem is increased, the individual may merely feel more happy and confident, or move to a euphoric state (formal disorder states such as 'mania' or 'hypomania' are not being considered here). If self-esteem is decreased, 'depression' can result. Self-esteem is decreased if there is exposure to a significant acute and/or chronic stressor, and/or when the individual's personality style causes psychotransmitter perturbations. Thus, vulnerabilities (shortly defined) ensure that the psychotransmitter locks onto and diminishes the individual's self-esteem rather than passing on by without any effect.

Table 7.1 Terms used in our model of 'psychotransmission'.

- *Self-esteem*, the key component of mood state and metaphorically akin to a biological 'gene' in terms of its end-point centrality to this model. We are euthymic when our self-esteem is maintained at a stable level, and are depressed when self-esteem drops. Positive fostering of self-esteem drives feelings of well-being, self-efficacy, and confidence. Conversely, negative provocation or 'switching off' of self-esteem can lead to depression.
- *Temperament* reflects here the innate excitability of the psychotransmission system (akin to neuronal function). For example, 'high neuroticism' may reflect the propensity of a neuron to discharge a psychological impulse at the slightest provocation.
- *Personality style* relates here to the way in which a 'neuron' registers psychotransmission from other 'neurons' (first messengers) and encodes any second messengers.
- A '*communication channel*', whether mediated by speech, letter-writing, or body language, is conceptualised as akin to the 'synaptic cleft', that is, the space between the two neurons through which psychotransmitter messages are passed from one neuron to the other. 'Message sent' by the initiator neuron may not be 'message received' at the receptor neuron.
- Messages are conveyed by *psychotransmission*, the analogy being that psychotransmitters capture the salient nuances of a stressor, and are stored in 'psychic packages' (vesicles), and eventually released when a stimulus (life event) is of sufficient severity, valency, and saliency.
- *Receptors*, the psychotransmitters are conceptualised as generally 'docking' on receptors. However, certain receptors may 'neutralise' the psychotransmitter, while others allow it to be further processed. Other receptors allow a 'key and lock' analogy (i.e. certain vulnerable receptors as 'locks' reflect early developmental factors, with psychotransmitters mimicking 'keys' in this instance) where the psychotransmitter locks onto the receptor and causes pathologically high levels of stimulation.
- '*Keys*' and '*locks*' are represented respectively by psychotransmitters and the receptors with which they 'dock'. The psychotransmitter 'key' represents the type of stimulus or stressor which, by itself, may not carry particular significance. The task of the receptor 'lock' is to prevent or allow docking (the interpretation and reaction to the psychotransmitter is dependent on the relevance of its characteristics) of the psychotransmitter. For example, people may or may not develop depression following a stressor mirroring events in earlier years.
- *Attributional and perceptual styles* are reflected in the attributIONal channels which open and close in response to the psychotransmitter-receptor (life events and their interpretation) complexes as well as second messengers and enzymes within the neuron (personality style).

Table 7.1 (*Continued*).

• Early learning experiences, exposure to aberrant parenting styles, experiences of trauma, and other developmental factors which shape *cognitive schemas* are analogous to intracellular enzymes, while *coping repertoires* and *defence mechanisms* are analogous to intracellular proteins. These elements facilitate the production of other messenger signals which ultimately 'switch on' or 'switch off' self-esteem. They may also have influenced neuronal development resulting in stunted neurons and setting up anomalous hard wiring circuits at a vulnerable neurodevelopmental stage, thus producing relatively fixed and inappropriately weighted circuits (e.g. favouring the 'self-critical' neuron).

Fig. 7.9 Our psycho-transmitter model.

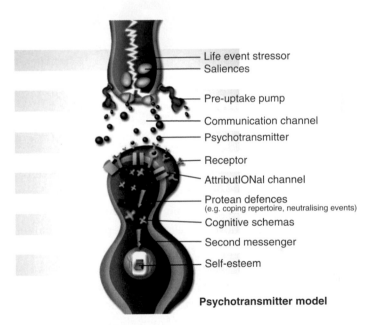

Life event stressor
Saliences
Pre-uptake pump
Communication channel
Psychotransmitter
Receptor
AttributIONal channel
Protean defences
(e.g. coping repertoire, neutralising events)
Cognitive schemas
Second messenger
Self-esteem

Psychotransmitter model

Salience of stressors may be determined at two points in our model. In the first, some stressors are deemed to be intrinsically salient to most people (e.g. death of a child) while others are salient only to some (e.g. negative evaluation by another). Salience may also be either trivial or profound. At the next level, the salience of a stressor emerges from personality style, coping repertoires and earlier life experiences where self-esteem may be sensitised and more prone to being lowered or turned off. Personality style dictates how the stressor is processed. If the personality style prevents the psychotransmitter from locking on to the receptor (via the pre-uptake pump

Fig. 7.10
Neurotransmitter and
psychotransmitter
models contrasted.

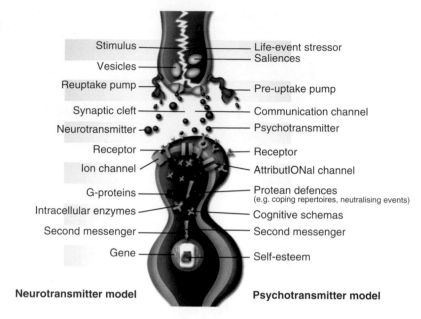

Neurotransmitter model	Psychotransmitter model
Stimulus	Life-event stressor
	Saliences
Vesicles	
Reuptake pump	Pre-uptake pump
Synaptic cleft	Communication channel
Neurotransmitter	Psychotransmitter
Receptor	Receptor
Ion channel	AttributIONal channel
G-proteins	Protean defences (e.g. coping repertoires, neutralising events)
Intracellular enzymes	Cognitive schemas
Second messenger	Second messenger
Gene	Self-esteem

or a range of other mechanisms), depression does not result. If it locks on to the receptor, but restitutive personality and coping repertoires (resilient second messenger systems) destroy, redirect or otherwise change the valency of the psychotransmitter, rapid remission occurs. If the second messenger systems are not resilient, an episode of non-melancholic depression is established – and if personality and coping repertoires do not (as second messenger systems) act to remove the valency of the psychotransmitter – then spontaneous remission is prevented and an episode of clinical non-melancholic depression is advanced. Contributing personality vulnerabilities also shape the clinical pattern of depressive symptoms and influence secondary coping mechanisms.

Our model for psychotransmission, as outlined above, provides a metaphorical illustration of how aetiological factors and risk factors may interact with personality style to promote the development of a non-melancholic depressive disorder. Clearly, we borrow from the chemical neurotransmission model. The latter may be viewed as hard science, as against our domain being viewed as fiction. However, we suggest that both can be considered as working models, designed to define process components that allow causes and pathology to be conceptualised. The chemical neurotransmission model has allowed a more 'rational' approach to the development of psychotropic drugs. Similarly, our psychotransmission model has the potential to clarify causes and pathogenesis at the system level. The model allows for considerations of treatment to be approached more logically, especially in determining where therapeutic 'leverage' could be applied. For instance, if the 'neuron' is intrinsically 'too excitable', a muting medication may be relevant. Conversely, if the problem relates to a 'key and lock' issue with a faulty attributIONal system, a cognitive behavioural approach may be relevant. In the same way that 'biological depression' is unlikely to be due solely to serotonin neurotransmission, as serotonin, noradrenaline, and dopaminergic neurons (and others) are involved in complex iterative circuits, we argue for a similar model for the multiple at-risk personality dimensions; that is, here we are also dealing with inter-dependent systems (Fig. 7.10).

In the subsequent chapters, this model will be used to further demonstrate how psychological and other interventions can play an important role in alleviating symptoms, addressing the causes and preventing the recurrence of such disorders. We first, however, consider each of the three components (self-esteem, personality style, and life event stressors) in some detail so as to prepare a logic for management strategies. As the aims of managing non-melancholic depression are to 'treat' the depression and to modulate predisposing variables so as to improve resilience, there is special benefit to defining system components and their contributing roles.

8

Self-esteem and self-worth in non-melancholic depression

As noted earlier, a depressed mood can be defined phenomenologically by three central features: feeling depressed, experiencing a drop in self-esteem, and feeling more self-critical. The third component is somewhat synonymous with a drop in self-esteem but also reflects the self-slighting and self-disparagement that occurs during a depressed mood, and evokes Freud's famous description of the shadow of the super-ego falling on the ego. It helps to explain why people who refuse to accept any personal limitations and find blame or fault with other people (e.g. paranoid individuals) rarely, if ever, get depressed because things that go wrong are always someone else's fault, not their own.

People clearly vary in terms of their level of self-esteem, but whatever its baseline level, it drops further during a depressed state and, even more importantly, it is the degree to which it drops that defines the severity of depression.

What are self-esteem and self-worth? Like all straightforward concepts, they have an ineffable component when we seek to define them. Self-esteem can be global in that the individual may rate him- or herself similarly on a whole range of attributes, or 'differentially' across a range of parameters. Thus, some people may see themselves as very worthwhile in a work context but, as they do not have a lot of close friends, view themselves as unlovable. Self-esteem can also be like Swiss cheese, solid in the main but with some big 'holes'. It is therefore not uncommon to see people who have a very high sense of self-esteem in most areas of their life but some selective self-esteem limitations (e.g. seeing themselves as intellectually 'dumb'), with such lacunae often reflecting developmental events, as detailed shortly in our description of the 'key and lock' model.

How does any individual obtain their self-esteem? We can only presume genetic and/or environmental influences. While it is unlikely that there is any gene or set of genes that dispose directly to 'self-esteem', we can suppose that those genes underpinning temperament and intrinsic personality characteristics, assemble a sense of 'self-concept', of 'me' and of 'identity', which have a value component, that is, the embryonic basis of such a sense of self-worth. Subsequently, developmental factors have the capacity to influence that embryonic state, both in terms of improving or stunting self-esteem, and influencing the extent to which it is preferentially internalised or externalised. For most children, parents are the most likely people to have such an influence. While there are many parental dimensions, the two principal constructs are ones of care, and overprotection or control (Parker, 1983). An intrinsically caring parent is affectionate, smiles a lot at the child, speaks in a warm and friendly voice and appears to understand the child's problems and worries. Parental care, as expressed across such constructs, generally leads to the child having a preferentially internalised self-esteem. For instance, if a baby or a child is playing on the floor and a parent walks by and gives them a hug and a smile, the child has to internalise that information ('Hey! I wasn't doing anything in particular but I got a big smile from my mum. I guess I must be likeable and loveable. I'll build on that'). In an ideal situation, parental care expressed over a sufficient period of time causes the child to incorporate such positive regard into a healthy level of internalised self-esteem. Lack of care – whether expressed by parents who are indifferent, distant, cold or more actively critical, rejecting, humiliating and abusive – predictably leads to a stunted sense of internalised self-esteem.

As noted, a second important dimension of parenting is overprotection or control. Here the parent is controlling, tends to intrude on the privacy of the child, imposes decisions rather than letting the child make their own decisions, can sometimes infantilise the child or make the child dependent on the parent, is often overprotective and makes the child feel as if they cannot look after themselves unless the parent is around. In less malignant situations, when the parent is 'good enough' in terms of caring, the impact on self-esteem may not be major, although the self-esteem is generally more externalised rather than internalised. The child is raised with stated or unstated injunctions such as 'If you eat all your green peas, you are a good boy' or 'If you make a mess on the floor, you are a bad boy'. Food is a common currency, with such parents often equating food as the care conduit. Thus, the child may receive harsher injunctions which carry implications ('If you love me you will eat all the green peas. If you do not eat all your food, that means you do not love me'). Such parenting evokes the wonderful image portrayed by Salinger (in a highly popular radio show in the USA: 'The Quiz Kids: The Eighth Day of Creation – Frannie and Zoey') of Mrs. Carpenter, who was described as cruising up and down her children's alimentary canal like a submarine. In such instances, the child's self-esteem is predictably externalised, so that they see themselves as only being 'good' (if that was the parents' emphasised value) if they have their clothes neat and tidy or all their work finished on time (if that was the parental emphasis). Not uncommonly, as adults they take up positions in organisations that value rules and procedures, and feel reasonably 'good' about themselves if they work to maintain those value systems. When asked to define themselves, self-descriptions usually invoke a weighting to such externalised values, and they have difficulty in defining their inner self. An overprotected child with an externalised self-esteem can often function comfortably in the home environment but, on leaving home or on taking up other independent tasks, can have predictable difficulties in adjusting to the differing 'rules of the game'. Thus, a child that has been exposed to an overprotective parent who praised them unconditionally (while still maintaining the umbilical cord) may feel quite empty when no longer the recipient of praise in their daily interactions with other meaningful people.

Parents are not the only figures that may shape an individual's self-esteem in the early years. The impact of siblings, peers, and teachers, as well as a range of life experiences, are well recognised. We assume then that early adverse life experiences result in distorted interpretations of events and beliefs about the world which, in turn, shape sensitivities and vulnerabilities within the individual's self-esteem, so determining their reaction to subsequent experiences. Lowered expectations, selective attention to failure, self-defeating behaviours and self-criticism are some of the many consequences of exposure to early adversity that influence the development of self-esteem (and personality style) and thus shape vulnerability to depressive disorders.

We can presume that, by late childhood or early adolescence, most individuals will have established their intrinsic level of self-esteem and self-worth, with their internalised or externalised weighting also reasonably established. But is self-esteem immutable and unmodifiable? Clinical observation and several longitudinal studies suggest, importantly, that self-esteem is modifiable to a significant degree. In one British study (Quinton & Rutter, 1984), the authors selected women who had been in a girls' home and who had clearly been deprived in their earlier years. Those who, on leaving the girls' home, and made a good marital choice, tended to have high levels of self-esteem, and were no more likely to develop depression than members of the general community. Those, by contrast, who married an individual who was critical, demeaning or non-supportive, had high levels of depression. We also undertook a study where we recruited a group of women and had them rate their parenting in their earliest years, as well as the level of care that they perceived from their husbands (Parker & Hadzi-Pavlovic, 1984). Those who received little care from both their fathers and their husbands had a very high rate of lifetime depression. Those who had received high care from both figures had a low rate of lifetime depression. Those who had been recipients of high parental care but who perceived their husbands as uncaring, had a lifetime rate of depression some 80% of the level held by those who experienced low care from both figures. Those who had received low paternal care, but then had a caring and affectionate husband, had a rate only slightly higher than those who had received care from both figures. Such data suggest that self-esteem is more likely to be influenced (for better or for worse) to a higher degree by more recent (albeit ongoing) influences rather than merely being the immutable inheritance of early events. This is clearly encouraging in arguing for the restitutive effects that can be effected and promoted by good psychotherapy and counselling, and by self-esteem-enhancing life events.

As noted earlier, self-esteem is central to our understanding of the nature of depression, and to non-melancholic depression in particular. Firstly, it assists in differentiating depression from anxiety and grief. Depression is a state marked by a drop in self-esteem. Anxiety, by contrast, is quintessentially a state of insecurity, uncertainty, apprehension, or fear. While depressed people are commonly anxious, and while high levels of anxiety drive depression, their frequent co-occurrence should not cause them to be viewed as synonymous, and it is important to differentiate them. Again, as noted earlier, in grief there is a sense of loss of something of value but no primary drop in self-esteem.

The second reason why the concept of self-esteem is central is that any vulnerability to depression is expressed across or via the domains in which we invest our self-esteem. For most people, self-esteem is principally invested in an intimate relationship but it can also be invested in work. Clearly, those who make a preferential investment in their partner, and whose partner is critical or who abandons them, are at particular risk. By contrast, the individual who invests their pride (i.e. a variant of self-esteem) in their work and who is criticised about their job performance or who is demoted or retrenched, is clearly then highly likely to be vulnerable to develop depression. Less common investments are observed clinically. For instance, some people who have never been able to develop a trusting relationship with another human being may make a major investment in a pet and develop a suicidal depression if their dog or cat dies. Other clinical nuances include the beautiful woman who invests her self-esteem in her beauty but, for whatever reason, asks a plastic surgeon to make some minor change. On recovery from the operation, she judges her persona as dramatically changed and develops a severe depression feeling that she has lost her sense of 'self' (true, to a degree), as her self-esteem is invested in her physical appearance.

Thus, our sense of self-esteem is the fulcrum to our mood state, both to states of depression and states of euphoria. We go through life and experience stressors on a daily basis. Whether varying from the severe to the mundane, they are unlikely to have much impact on our mood unless they influence our self-esteem. Here the concept of attributional style (part of the 'secondary messenger system') is of relevance. Life events do not, by themselves, necessarily induce depression. It is the perception of the life event that is all-important. Thus, the event of a woman walking out on her husband would generally be viewed as a significant life event. The husband's interpretation, however, is far more salient than the actual event. If he interprets that he has failed again, and that he has no capacity to ever maintain a loving relationship as a consequence of all his intrinsic flaws, he is likely to develop depression. If, by contrast, he processes the event by saying 'Great! She's gone ... I never liked her anyway', it is unlikely that he will develop depression. As Beck et al. (1979) note in an overview chapter to their book on cognitive behaviour therapy, Epicetetus, a Greek philosopher of the 1st century, commented: 'Men are disturbed not by things but by the views which they take of them'.

As self-esteem is the mood 'fulcrum', we also enjoy events and interactions that increase our self-esteem. While many examples could be chosen, the wedding ceremony is probably a quintessential experience. While clearly a rite of passage, weddings have potential secondary benefits, in that the couple is the centre of attention and the recipient of goodwill, generosity of spirit and fine words that attest to their individual strengths. If the wedding ceremony and reception proceed with such an emphasis, it would be difficult to imagine an individual not having their self-esteem rise and for the wedding to be remembered for a lengthy period. For a couple who love each other, the ceremony reinforces that emotional commitment and, as their self-esteem's investment in the other is enhanced, there is a secondary benefit to their own level of self-esteem.

Any individual's self-esteem can be enhanced (or diminished) by a range of broader and less individualised social events, and sport serves as a good example. When an Australian yacht won the America's Cup for the first time after many attempts and decades of trying, the effects on the community were noteworthy. People going to work smiled, waved and blew their car horns at each other. The Prime Minister of the day captured the euphoria and the national self-esteem in criticising any employer who did not allow an employee to take the day off. Watching the successes (and failures) of the Australian Rugby Union Wallaby team in the last few decades reveals similar effects. In 'esteemed' events (e.g. Rugby World Cup, Test Matches) and when playing high-ranking international teams and, particularly, winning in the last few minutes, the average Australian Rugby tragic sitting in the stadium exemplifies the impact of 'winning' on individual, communal, and national self-esteem. People feel good about the result and about themselves. They show a generosity of spirit, they talk more and often more loudly, they may sing while those around them are most likely to be seen as their best mates – as having shared in some primitive ritual and, in overcoming the odds, their self-esteem has inflated. In extreme instances, we remember the apocryphal South American vignette where one fanatical soccer follower said that if his national team were to win the World Cup he would be so thrilled that he would kill himself. The team did and he did.

9

Personality style and functioning as a contributor to non-melancholic depression

Introduction

'It is more important to know what sort of person has a disease, than to know what sort of disease has a person'.

–Hippocrates (460–370 BC)

Many years ago Kiloh et al. (1972) suggested that non-melancholic depression 'may well be dimensional, encompassing a number of ways in which patients can mobilise their defence mechanisms to cope with environmental and intra-psychic threats'. Such a model encompasses two components: *life event stressors*, as well as *personality and coping repertoires*. In this section, we report on our studies assessing the relevance of personality as:

(i)   increasing the risk to depression,
(ii) shaping the phenotypic picture (or clinical pattern) of the non-melancholic disorders,
(iii) influencing treatment response.

Over time, personality style is likely to shape one's lifestyle and immediate environment, which, in turn, may either directly or indirectly influence

---

Propositions

Personality style influences:
- Vulnerability to depressive episodes.
- Exposure to lifestyle and environmental stressors.
- Symptom patterns of non-melancholic depressive episodes.
- Coping responses to the stressor and to the depressed state.
- Response to differing treatments.

the level of exposure to certain types of stressors, so that the iterations between predispositional personality factors and triggering life event stressors can be observed.

We use the term 'personality' to also encompass 'temperament', allowing that the two are viewed as synonymous by many, while worthy of distinction by others. For those who distinguish the two, 'temperament' is more likely to be viewed as the 'hard-wiring' that underpins expression of certain behavioural characteristics, while 'personality' is the end state of developmental factors, as well as of social and cultural influences, impinging on 'temperament'. The distinction is of considerable importance theoretically as it allows the possibility that some individuals may be destined to develop non-melancholic depression largely as a consequence of their 'temperament' and presumably as a consequence of genetic factors rather than as a consequence of developmental factors (e.g. lack of parental care, abuse) that are commonly imputed as 'real world' social determinants. In practice, clarification of any such distinction is limited, and we therefore use the term 'personality' to refer to both determining domains, allowing that some of the identified personality dimensions may be entirely or largely 'hard wired' while others may reflect interaction of both genetic and environmental influences.

As suggested in the chapter title, we consider both personality style and personality functioning. The argument for considering the latter benefits from a brief explanation. Many studies seeking to identify separate depressive classes or types, have imputed the relevance of 'personality disorder' (PD). For instance, Paykel (1971) undertook a cluster analysis of a large sample of depressed patients and, in his four-cluster solution, identified a group labelled as 'Young depressives with personality disorder'. The problems in measuring PD are multiple and well recognised. The most appropriate model (categorical versus dimensional) has not been resolved, response biases and rating difficulties lead to low reliability, while individuals meeting criteria for one disorder tend to meet criteria for 4–6 other disorders, and with such 'co-morbidity' building to further imprecision. We suggest that a contribution to such confounding emerges from having diagnostic criteria for PDs that are an admixture of descriptors of personality style and of functioning. The ubiquitous presence of one component of functioning across separate disorder classes can then generate co-morbidity, independent of the principal objective to capture separate styles. For instance, most of the currently classified PDs have criteria that assess 'impulsiveness' to some degree (with it being generally increased in the so-called Cluster B conditions, and generally decreased in the Cluster C disorders). Such non-specificity leads to difficulties then in distinguishing separate PDs. We will therefore shortly report on a study (Parker et al., 2004) where we modelled disordered functioning independent of style.

General model of personality

Our research sought to identify the personality styles that might predispose to non-melancholic depression. We adopted two strategies, examining both 'general' models of personality and also (using clinical observation) identifying personality styles seemingly over-represented in our non-melancholic depressed patients. Each approach is now reported in brief.

One (the so-called Eysenkian model) emphasises two key dimensions: extraversion and neuroticism. The extreme end of the extroversion dimension represents the propensity of an individual to seek novelty, avoid routine and crave stimulation and company. Introversion, at the other extreme of the dimension, is represented by the desire to seek routine and to avoid change. 'Neuroticism', in this model, refers to levels of autonomic arousal, rather than to a character style of being 'neurotic'. Individuals high on 'neuroticism' are viewed as being more likely to be highly reactive to stress, and to be tense and nervy, while those low on this dimension tend to be more phlegmatic and relaxed in their approach to life.

For the last decade at least, and building on a lengthy research history, the broader North American Five-Factor Model (or FFM) (Costa & McCrae, 1990) has been widely accepted as a model of principal personality dimensions. The FFM evolved from several theories of personality, the most influential being Cattell's in the 1940s, which used factor analysis to refine the study of personality traits. Its final form resulted from extensive factor analyses of several personality tests and scales (McCrae & Costa, 1985) and represents an inductive approach to the study of personality (i.e. that the theory has emerged from research data). This model advocates the use of the same dimensions applied across individuals, and its constructs, which are described below, have been replicated in several independent (including cross-cultural) studies of personality. The FFM constructs of personality are:

- neuroticism versus emotional stability,
- introversion versus extraversion,
- conscientiousness versus fecklessness,
- agreeableness versus cold-heartedness and hostility,
- imagination and openness to experience versus being traditional and set in one's ways.

We pursued how well the dimensions in this latter model correspond to styles that we observe in our non-melancholic depressed patients. Our clinical observation suggests that an anxious worrying style is the most commonly observed personality style (at least in those with non-melancholic depression), a style quite similar (but less pejorative in labelling) to the FFM construct of 'neuroticism'. Secondly, we see shy and behaviourally inhibited subjects, corresponding to the FFM 'introversion' construct. Thirdly, we see obsessional and perfectionistic individuals (corresponding to the FFM 'conscientiousness' construct), who deconstruct when attempting to deal with certain stressors (usually involving an inability to control a situation). Fourthly, we see irritable and hostile non-melancholic patients, as identified in many multivariate studies (e.g. Matussek et al., 1982), consistent with the less 'agreeable' FFM personality construct, whether they express it in an on-going way or only in response to stress. Finally, we see those who have historically been described as having a 'characterological depression', and who often state that have been depressed from birth (and which might then suggest a predisposition emerging more from low-self-esteem rather than from a personality style). Thus, approximation of four of the constructs to the FFM model encouraged our initial studies, which clearly pursued an unstated hypothesis that extremes in 'normal' personality or temperament dimensions increase the risk to depression and, in particular, to non-melancholic depression.

We pursued this model in one study and, seeking to overcome any referral biases that might shape a psychiatric sample, we studied a sample of more than 600 general practitioner patients (Parker & Roy, 2002). Just over half responded positively to a probe question assessing a lifetime episode of 'depression' and with half of those having had episodes that were likely to have been clinical depression. For those reporting any lifetime episode, one-half of them had consulted a general practitioner and one-quarter a psychiatrist, while one-fifth of the whole sample had previously received an antidepressant.

Separate multivariate analyses argued against a categorical model for the personality dimensions. Dimensional analyses (i.e. factor analysis) favoured a 6-factor solution. While the first general factor contained both *'anxious worrying'* and *'irritability'* items (corresponding to the FFM construct of 'neuroticism' or emotional instability), when a final 6-factor solution was imposed, those two separated as factors, albeit with scores showing a modest correlation. In addition to the 'irritability' dimension, our 6-factor solution identified a *'self-centredness'* dimension, with component 'hostile, volatile, and entitled' features perhaps corresponding to the FFM construct of low 'agreeableness', and with scores on this dimension being modestly associated with scores on the irritability dimension. Such results allowed some theoretical speculation. We suggested then that those with high-trait anxiety either internalise their anxiety (by anxious worrying) or, alternatively, externalise it via irritability (being crabby, snappy, and hot-tempered). By contrast, those who have a 'hostile depression' appear more likely to have a Cluster B personality style (and score high on self-centredness), and are more likely to respond to stress and depression by acting out impulsively and with volatility. The remaining factors were labelled '*introversion*', '*obsessionality*', and '*self-blame*', with the first two corresponding closely to FFM constructs of introversion and conscientiousness.

Multivariate analyses examined the extent to which scores on each factor were associated with depression variables. High 'anxious worrying' scores were predictive of all depression outcome variables (state depression severity, lifetime depression, receipt of professional help, and prescription of antidepressant medication). Higher irritability, self-blame, and introversion scores (and lower obsessionality scores) made an additional (and minor) independent contribution to only some depression variables, while self-centredness scores were quite unrelated to any depression variable. Our study therefore identified styles associated with (i) increased risk (i.e. anxious worrying, irritability, and self-blame), (ii) decreased risk (i.e. obsessionality), and (iii) no risk (i.e. self-centredness) to depression onset.

Results therefore further suggested the key relevance of an 'anxious worrying' personality style as a risk factor to depression. In an earlier study (Parker et al., 1998a) we had also identified the prominence of an 'anxious worrying' personality style in those who develop non-melancholic depression. Such patients also had high levels of state anxiety during their depressive episode, building to the 'spectrum' model (linking personality and clinical features), that we will detail shortly. Background history suggested a strong genetic component to their anxiety. Thus, they were more likely to have had a parent who had had an anxiety disorder, more likely to show behavioural inhibition and school refusal in their younger years, more likely to have a Cluster C personality style, scored high on measures of trait anxiety and worrying, and, in comparison to other subjects, developed their disorder at a younger age, as well as having more frequent and lengthier depressive episodes. Thus, we suggested that a genetically underpinned 'anxious worrying' temperament style both increased the risk to depression and, in reaction to a life event stressor, amplified those anxiety features, to shape a phenotypic picture of 'anxious depression'.

Similarly, we suggested that those who scored high on the personality measure of 'irritability' had high levels of externalised anxiety, with their anxiety again increasing their risk to depression. When seen clinically, such patients are generally 'nice' and 'agreeable' people, who are almost invariably guilty about being snappy to family members, and seemingly not warranting descriptors such as 'hostile' or disagreeable.

But how can we reconcile high scores on the obsessional factor being linked to a decreased risk of depression and of receiving professional treatment with clinical experience? Firstly, while clinicians see individuals with distinctly obsessional personality styles that does not mean, of necessity, that such a style increases the general risk of depression in the community. We reason that highly obsessional individuals are less likely to expose themselves to depressogenic stressors and, if they do become depressed, are less likely to admit to it or wish to seek help, so contributing to the negative associations with our depression variables. However, those who come to clinical attention have commonly deconstructed, having particularly bleak views about the future, seeing no options for proceeding and describing considerable guilt. Secondly, there may be differences between being 'obsessional' and being 'perfectionistic', and we therefore thought it useful to pursue the latter concept in a subsequent study.

Again, while those high on self-centredness are commonly observed clinically, our failure to find support for this personality style as a risk factor was interpreted as such individuals being disposed to diffuse their depression by externalised hostility which is useful to that individual (though associated with considerable collateral damage to those around).

As the FFM temperament models do not include a self-blame dimension, it was not clear whether our self-blame factor reflected the intrusion of a 'state depression' factor, or whether it captured the clinical description of 'characterological depression'. If 'self-blame' was neither state depression nor a 'normal' personality (qua temperament) dimension, we assume that it reflects the impact of early developmental stressors (e.g. critical, judgmental, or demeaning experiences) and the development of a self-blaming cognitive set, but whether this is best modelled as a 'personality' construct or as a 'low-self-esteem' construct is problematic.

Following the testing of the relevance of a general model of personality, we initiated a refined study. Here we pursued whether 'perfectionism' might be a more useful construct than 'obsessionality', as perfectionists tend to set unrealistic standards and, at times, feel that they have failed, self-blame and judge themselves as inadequate, and so risk depression. We expanded the 'self-blame' item set. We also elected to consider two expressions of introversion: one emphasising *social shyness* and the other focusing more on *personal reserve* in close relationships. We also pursued the utility of two other personality styles that appear conceptually to be independent of the FFM model (apart from 'neuroticism') but which are also observed clinically in those who develop non-melancholic depression. In an earlier study (Boyce & Parker, 1989) we had identified 'interpersonal rejection sensitivity' as a stronger predictor to post-natal depression than neuroticism, and it is a key construct to the Diagnostic and Statistical Manual of Mental Disorders (DSM-IV) definition of 'atypical depression'. Secondly, Beck (1983) defined a 'sociotropic' style as exerting a high risk to depression via the needs of the sociotropic individual to please and rely on others, and so, when stressed or faced with the loss of the other, being highly vulnerable to depression.

Our 89-item Temperament and Personality (T&P) questionnaire (comprising items designed to measure eight a priori constructs) was initially completed by another sample of 529 patients (aged 16–70 years; 56% being female) while waiting to see their general practitioner. Exploratory factor analyses favoured an 8-factor model, and using the highest loading items on each factor, we then created 8 scales, labelled: *'anxious worrying'*, *'perfectionism'*, *'personal reserve'*, *'irritability'*, *'social avoidance'*, *'self-focused'* (or low understanding of others), *'self-criticism'*, and *'sensitivity to rejection'* (see Table 9.1). The respective percentage variances accounted for were: 20.0%, 8.7%, 6.7%, 4.7%, 3.3%, 2.4%, 2.2%, and 1.9% (totalling 50%). The internal consistency of the scales ranged from 0.62 to 0.91 (mean 0.84). The great majority of the items defined in the factors and contributing to the respective scales emerged from their a priori construct status (including all 11 of the 'perfectionism' items, all 9 of the 'personal reserve', all 9 of the 'social avoidance', all 11 of the 'irritability', and all 4 of the 'self-criticism' items).

Scale scores for our sample were then compared in a preliminary study against scale scores returned by a series of depressed out-patients to determine the extent to which scales might differentiate the two groups. The depressed patients returned significantly higher scores on six of the eight scales (most distinctly for 'anxious worrying', followed by 'self-criticism', 'sensitivity to rejection', 'social avoidance', 'personal reserve', and 'irritability').

Table 9.1 The eight personality styles identified as relevant to non-melancholic depression.

Externalising styles	Internalising styles
Irritability	Anxious worrying
Self-focused	Self-criticism
	Personal reserve
	Social avoidance
	Perfectionism
	Sensitivity to rejection

Trends for the depressed subjects to score higher on the 'perfectionism' and on 'self-focused' scales were not formally significant.

Formal tests of the properties of our T&P questionnaire are proceeding, as well as studies pursuing our central hypothesis – that these dimensions reflect risk to onset and/or persistence of non-melancholic depression, relate to treatment adherence and influence differential treatment-modality responses. Appendix 3 describes our T&P questionnaire and provides information about its psychometric properties.

It is possible (see Table 9.1) to aggregate the eight identified dimensions into 'externalising' and 'internalising' constructs in response to stress. An 'externalising' style may be assumed to subsume a temperament style characterised by high levels of autonomic arousal and irritability, whereby individuals are disposed to be more likely to 'blow up' when upset and engage in reckless or impulsive behaviours when depressed. As discussed, this style may dispose to increased episodes of depression, but (as a consequence of externalising the stress) such individuals are more likely to experience only transient-depressive episodes, although others around them may experience 'collateral' damage as a consequence of the individual's response style.

By contrast, internalisers are more likely to 'stew' on events and seek activities that distract them from their worries when depressed. An 'internalising' style subsumes personality features of anxious worrying, being self-critical, being shy or reserved, being socially avoidant, perfectionistic, and sensitivity to rejection by others. Individuals with these broad behavioural responses tend to have high levels of self-blame and pessimistic thinking (interspersed with feelings of guilt and remorse over the pain they may have caused others), so increasing the likelihood of experiencing episodes of depression, and more prolonged episodes. We assume that stress exaggerates such dispositional personality features, so that those who are prone to worry will become even more worry-bound to the extent of inactivity; those who tend to be perfectionists may become paralysed by the anxiety associated with making a possible wrong decision; and those that have an emotional 'hair trigger' response style are more likely to become volatile and critical of those around them.

How well does our model correspond to the FFM? The NEO-PI-R (Revised NEO Personality Inventory) was developed by Costa and McCrae (1992) as an FFM measure and it is possible to cross-match our eight identified constructs. Thus, the NEO construct of neuroticism has facets akin to our identified dimensions of anxious worrying, irritability, self-criticism, and sensitivity to rejection. The NEO construct of introversion has constructs akin to our identified dimensions of personal reserve and social avoidance.

The-8 factor model for temperament and personality styles in non-melancholic depression

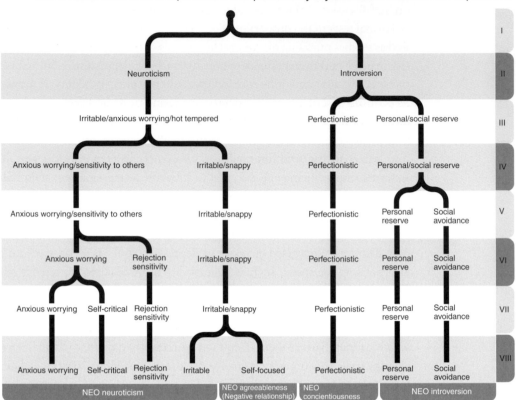

Fig. 9.1 The 8-factor model and its relationship to the NEO model.

NEO conscientiousness corresponds to our construct of perfectionism, and the NEO construct of agreeableness corresponds (negatively) to our self-focused construct (see Fig. 9.1).

Figure 9.1 was developed by modelling a series of factor analyses on responses to our T&P questionnaire among a sample of 903 adults who responded to our online web-based survey and who had suffered from an episode of unipolar depression. Factor numbers were restricted at each analysis running from 2-factor to 8-factor solutions, to demonstrate how higher-order constructs have sub-sets and how they arborise to lower order constructs. It is of interest to note how early (i.e. at the 2-factor level) 'perfectionism' emerges from a higher-order 'introversion' construct and how it remains quite 'pure' across the differing levels. The remaining personality styles have their origins in a 'neuroticism' factor (also evident in the 2-factor solution). At the 4-factor solution level, we have a model very similar to the FFM, with correspondence to the NEO: NEO neuroticism equates to 'stress/worry'; NEO agreeableness equates to 'irritable/hot-tempered'; NEO extraversion equates (inversely) to 'social/personal reserve/inhibition'; and NEO conscientiousness equates to 'perfectionistic'. However, we have elected to pursue the relevance of the 8-factor model as there may be aetiological and treatment gradient differences between those who rate differently on the 'anxious worrying', 'rejection sensitivity' and 'self-critical' dimensions (as against the higher-order construct) as there may be for those who score differently on the 'personal reserve' and 'social inhibition' dimensions.

Our 'self-focused' factor, while related to our 'irritability' factor, stands alone as representing the NEO construct of (negative) agreeableness. Clinically, this factor appears related more to disordered functioning than reflecting personality style. In our model, the 'self-focused' factor is related to that of irritability possibly through the construct of 'impulsivity'.

In an important article, Livesley et al. (1998) undertook a number of analyses examining the utility of the FFM to modelling disordered personality and with genetic analyses supporting four of the five FFM dimensions, with an accompanying editorial of Widiger (1998) appropriately titled (there and in this instance) that 'Four Out of Five Ain't Bad'. At the 4-factor solution in our analyses, the same constructs were identified. Thus, to the extent that these four dimensions are relevant to a general model of personality, and genetically underpinned, then they may be viewed as dimensions of temperament. It then becomes appropriate to hypothesise that such temperament dimensions dispose those who have high scores to non-melancholic depression. We doubt, on the theoretical basis, that non-melancholic depression reflects genetic destiny but some personality-based 'hard-wiring' contribution could well be assumed.

While most studies seeking to identify 'genes' for major depression have proved disappointing, our sub-typing model would argue for considering quite differing genetic influences contributing to melancholic and to non-melancholic depressive disorders, and, for the latter, with the genes operating at the personality (rather than at the depressive) level.

Personality functioning

As noted earlier, current limitations to diagnosing and measuring the PDs encouraged a study designed to model and measure disordered personality function. Our model was encouraged by a quote from Millon and Davis (1996) in regard to the PDs: 'Perhaps the word diagnosis can be eventually dispensed with, in favour simply of assessment of functioning'. Measuring personality style and disordered function independently has the capacity to clarify whether most or all PD personality styles are associated non-specifically with disordered function, or whether each personality style shapes specific manifestations of disordered functioning. Currently, the DSM-IV and the International Classification of Diseases (ICD-10) criteria for the PDs emphasise personality traits, although as traits may be intrinsically maladaptive, or only maladaptive above a certain imprecise threshold or in specific contexts, such an emphasis effectively avoids the reality that assessing *functioning* may be more salient.

We assembled – via a lengthy review (Parker et al., 2004) of relevant literature, a set of constructs that suggested disordered personality functioning:

(i)   disagreeableness,
(ii)   inflexibility,
(iii)   being uncaring to others,
(iv)   lack of empathy,
(v)   being ineffective,
(vi)   having a self-defeating life pattern,
(vii)   failing to learn from experience,
(viii) being impulsive,
(ix)   being pessimistic,
(x)   immorality,
(xi)   being unstable under stress,
(xii)   lacking self-direction,
(xiii) non-cooperativeness,
(xiv)   causing discomfort to others,
(xv)   maladaptability,
(xvi)   failure to form and maintain relationships,
(xvi)   lack of humour.

A large set of self-reported descriptors of those constructs were factor analysed in a sample of patients with clinician-diagnosed personality dysfunction and comparisons made with control samples.

Results (Parker et al., 2004) suggested a far more parsimonious model of disordered personality functioning than anticipated – comprising two higher-order constructs underpinned by limitations in 'co-operativeness' and in 'coping' – and with the model being linked to all PD personality styles (rather than having narrow application to only certain PD styles). The co-operativeness dimension was underpinned by items suggesting care and concern about others, being good-hearted, ready to lend an ear, flexibility in thought and action, and both being able to connect readily with other people and being able to understand the other person's point of view.

The coping dimension was defined by coping and succeeding, by having the capacity to organise oneself and think before acting, to be able to size up situations and not over-react to minor frustrations in life, and to learn from mistakes that had been made. A set of validation studies indicated that those with a PD scored distinctly lower on both dimensions, but with differentiation being driven more by limitations in co-operativeness than by limitations in coping.

There is historical support for such a parsimonious model, with Freud (see Erikson, 1995) defining full maturity as requiring only two markers: 'Lieben und arbeiten' (to love and to work) (p 238). 'To love' was assumed to refer to the capacity to make and maintain intimate relationships, and assumes co-operation. 'To work' referred not merely to being employable but involved in 'work-productiveness'. The centrality of 'co-operativeness' has been emphasised previously. For example, Livesley et al. (1998) defined PD as reflecting a tripartite failure of (i) the self-system, with failure to establish stable and integrated representation of self and others; (ii) adaptive function in interpersonal relationships; and (iii) prosocial and co-operative relationships, while Rutter (1987) observed that 'a pervasive persistent abnormality in maintaining social relationships' underpinned many of the categorised PDs. In terms of coping, several writers (e.g. Kruedelbach et al., 1993; Vollrath et al., 1998) have argued for a coping paradigm for modelling disordered personality function. Again, Livesley et al. (1998) emphasised inflexibility and inadequate performance in 'the universal life tasks of identity, attachment, intimacy, and affiliation'. Finally, and although we adopted a 'bottom up' approach in assembling putative constructs, our two-construct model is similar to that proposed by Cloninger, with one study by his group (Svrakic et al., 1993) identifying character scale scores of low 'self-directedness' and low 'co-operativeness' as highly discriminating of those with and without a PD.

Such results encourage a research model testing the utility of a two-tiered model of PD which might first measure the likelihood of disordered personality function (e.g. 'definite', 'probable', 'possible', and 'absent') and, secondarily, measure personality style – whether style constructs reflect normal dimensions or are weighted to prototypic PD styles. Such a model has the additional advantage of conceptually overcoming dysjunctions observed in clinical practice, where for instance, we observe patients who are successful as a consequence of their personality style (say sociopathic), and thus who score high on the personality style component but low on disordered functioning (i.e. 'successful' sociopathy) as against those who are 'failed sociopaths', and who would score high on both of the style and functioning components. The model clearly allows the impact of each axis to be calibrated.

Clearly, we argue that individuals low on the personality function domains of co-operativeness and coping are at greater risk of developing non-melancholic depression and also of having more persistent episodes, but such assertions await further quantification in applied studies of our measure.

The spectrum model

As noted earlier, we presuppose that certain neurobiological processes shape personality style, which, in turn, is accentuated when the individual is stressed or depressed and which influences the clinical features or phenotypic picture of the non-melancholic disorder. One such example of such a 'spectrum model' (i.e. atypical depression) has been described for an extensive period, with DSM-IV criteria amalgamating personality (e.g. rejection sensitivity) and clinical features (i.e. mood reactivity, appetite and weight gain, hypersomnia, and leaden paralysis). Our initial studies pursuing the utility of such a 'spectrum model' suggested three possible expressions within the non-melancholic domain: 'anxious worrying', 'irritable', and, less clearly, a 'hostile' depression. In a later study, we included items that might better be viewed as coping repertoires or homoeostatic mechanisms, as a consequence of pursuing the construct of 'atypical depression'. In that study (Parker et al., 2002a), we remodelled the DSM-IV features to suggest that the personality style of 'interpersonal rejection sensitivity' contributed to the development of 'anxiety' (principally social phobia and panic disorder). When individuals with such personality traits became depressed, we suggested that some features may more be homoeostatic mechanisms or coping repertoires rather than symptoms. Thus, the hypersomnia has a stress-reducing propensity, while appetite increase (more specifically, food cravings) is usually selective and focused on foods rich in certain peptides and the forerunners of L-tryptophan, allowing the homoeostatic interpretation.

It seemed useful to pursue such a broader model and, we therefore had a sample of non-melancholic subjects complete our earlier measure (albeit with limited domains) of personality style, and complete a sheet recording symptoms and coping responses generally engaged in when depressed. In this study (Parker et al., 2002b), evidence of relative specificity was demonstrated. Thus, those high on 'anxious worrying' were highly likely to be anxious when depressed and have an increased need for reassurance; those high on 'irritability' became distinctly more irritable and were distinctly more likely to seek pleasure; those high on 'social inhibition' were selectively more likely to withdraw socially; while those high on 'self-centredness' were

Fig. 9.2 Our spectrum model of non-melancholic depression linking personality style with clinical symptoms.

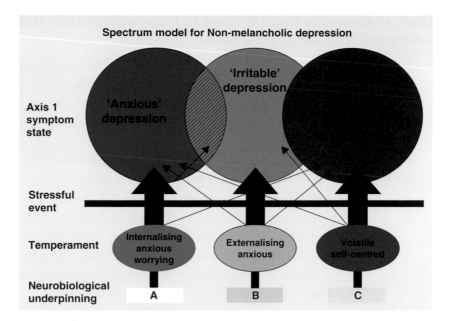

selectively more likely to be reckless, break things, spend money, and increase both alcohol and cigarette intake. These three examples of 'spectrum' disorders are illustrated again in Figure 9.2.

We propose to use our more comprehensive measure of personality style to examine the capacity of a spectrum model to be extended in breadth and enriched in depth. In combination with treatment studies, there is then the capacity to determine whether differing interventions act on the surface picture (i.e. symptoms, coping responses) or on underlying contributory personality components, an outcome which would further advance the utility of the 'spectrum' concept.

There is an additional advantage to the spectrum model. Just as we argued that the presence of observable psychomotor disturbance (PMD) in a depressed individual would argue for melancholic or psychotic depression, the clinician can use the 'clinical pattern phenotype' to advance aetiological and management decisions. Thus, the patient who presents with a non-melancholic depression but who essentially reports anxiety features as prominent may be more likely to have high-trait anxiety and to benefit from anxiety reduction management strategies as well as antidepressant ones. By contrast, the 'hostile' patient reporting a non-melancholic depression is unlikely to be very compliant with management, while the perfectionistic patient is likely to be resistant (despite being adherent) to many therapeutic interventions. Such nuances are extended in the next section.

Does personality contribution to non-melancholic depression influence treatment response?

As there is currently no accepted model for conceptualising differing expressions of non-melancholic depression, evidence of treatment specificity is lacking, although there are some interesting indicative data. In one study (Parker & Roy, 2002), we overviewed evidence suggesting that 'anxious depression' is highly likely (and 'irritable depression' quite likely) to respond to selective serotonin reuptake inhibitors (SSRI) antidepressants. That is, not only do people with such personality traits commonly report their depression as responding to an SSRI, but they also report lower levels of anxiety and that they 'worry' less. We suggest that both styles reflect a construct of 'emotional dysregulation' and that the SSRIs settle or mute that dysregulation and the associated anxiety. Thus, when an individual with non-melancholic depression reports significant lifetime high-trait anxiety we are optimistic about their likelihood of responding to an SSRI, and we detail later (in the application of the psychotransmitter model) how such medication influences the 'innate excitability' of the psychotransmitter neuron.

By contrast, those with an obsessional and perfectionistic personality style appear unlikely to show a distinct response to antidepressant medication or to the psychotherapies (Zuroff et al., 2000). Shahar et al. (2003) suggested that results reflected perfectionistic individuals being less satisfied with social relationships and therefore making little contribution to the therapeutic alliance. If valid, perfectionism might be presumed to mitigate against a therapeutic alliance by counteracting the impact of non-specific therapeutic ingredients that are recognised to contribute to remission. Our review (Parker et al., 1998a) suggested also that those with a 'hostile depression' have long been viewed (e.g. Blashfield & Morey, 1970) as unlikely to show improvement with any drug therapy, including tricyclic and neuroleptic medications. These data are only indicative but illustrate the important possibility that personality style has a major potential to influence response to differing drug and non-drug therapies for those with non-melancholic depression. This therefore argues strongly against any approach (be it drug or a psychotherapy) as having universal application to treating the non-melancholic disorders and leads to the specificity model that underpins the management chapters later in this book.

10

Stress as a contributor to non-melancholic depression

As noted in Chapter 1, the binary model of depression viewed one 'type' of depression (i.e. reactive or neurotic depression) as essentially being a response to a major or salient life-event stressor. By contrast, the other type of depression (endogenous or melancholic) was seen as a condition that occurred without any such trigger, with the term 'endogenous' emphasising that the depression came from 'within' rather than from stressors and the environment. We now turn to examine the role of life event stressors in those with non-melancholic disorders. Life event stressors may, theoretically, be all-explanatory and contribute totally to the onset of the depressive disorder. Terms such as 'reactive depression' and 'adjustment disorder with depressed mood' emphasise the contribution of a life event and do not recognise any predisposing or other factor. While life events may vary in their magnitude, one could posit that most of these 'pure state' reactions are likely to be in response to cataclysmic or extremely severe depressing events, and where it might be imagined that most people would develop such a depressive condition.

In many ways, these reactions are extensions of 'normal depression'. Studies of non-clinical groups suggest that most people experience depressed moods following relevant triggering events but that, for most these states last only minutes, hours, or days. Thus, most human beings experience a spontaneous remission of such moods with the mood state self-remitting, either naturally or in response to some (presumed) positive outcome. An analogy to Hook's law is relevant here. This law suggests that something can be stretched and expected to return to its normal shape under most circumstances. If, however, it is stretched too far, elasticity is lost. Pursuing the analogy, we can view these reactive disorders as being generally understandable and short-lived responses to life event stressors that have lowered the individual's self-esteem. But, if particularly severe and/or repeated, such reactivity may not spontaneously improve and may dispose the individual to a more chronic depressive disorder, and here use of the term 'reactive depression' no longer seems appropriate.

Shortly, we will argue for salience, as against severity, being the more commonly relevant construct for considering acute reactive disorders.

The 'learned helplessness' model (Seligman, 1972) has some utility for understanding the impact of chronic or persistent life event stressors. Unpredictability and uncontrollability are the two central components of 'learned helplessness'. The theory of the genesis of learned helplessness relies strongly on how animals (and humans) associate certain stimuli and behaviours with rewards and others with punishment or non-reinforcement. Laboratory evidence concerning the development of learned helplessness found that when an animal experienced a trauma it could not control, its motivation to respond in the face of later trauma waned. Even if it did respond to such later trauma, and the response succeeded in producing relief, the animal had trouble learning, perceiving, and believing that the response worked. Deficits in motivation found in animals that have undergone the learned helplessness procedure result in behaviours that mimic some types of depressive disorders in humans, particularly the more chronic non-melancholic disorders.

Much has been written about early adversity and the later development of depressive disorders. As noted earlier, we have argued for a 'key and lock' hypothesis for understanding how some people are particularly likely to develop a depressive condition in response to certain events (Parker et al., 1998b; Parker et al., 2000). Early life experiences, including early adversity, can shape the way in which a young child understands and perceives the world, makes sense of his own feelings and learns to trust and relate to adults. Our 'key and lock' hypothesis holds that certain early acute or chronic adverse experiences establish 'locks' or specific templates around the course and outcome of specific events, and which lay down a sensitivity to later mirroring events. Such adverse experiences create core vulnerabilities which may serve to increase the likelihood of exposure to further adverse experiences, yet with minimal resources for coping, some of which dispose the individual to develop depression in response to a 'mirroring' life event in adulthood, and which, operate as 'keys' and open the lock to depression. While early adverse experiences may establish non-specific vulnerability to depression (e.g. parenting experiences giving the child an intrinsically low self-esteem), the 'key and lock' hypothesis refers to 'specific' vulnerabilities, whereby certain events in childhood predispose the individual to depression when the earlier event is re-created. Thus, we argue that the salience (or special meaning to the individual) of an event (whether reflecting a personality influence on appraisal of the event or a 'key and lock' sequence) is often more important than the event's objective severity. Models of how the 'key and lock' sequence might operate are detailed in our psychotransmitter model.

There are several possible mechanisms whereby 'locks' are established. One possibility is that vulnerabilities set up by early adverse life experiences are mediated by specific sets of cognitions or 'schemas', with subsequent events processed according to attributional sets. Schemas are core beliefs that dictate our interpretation of the world and events, and may be expressed through expectations. Schemas are essentially unconditional and extremely resistant to change. Individuals who have not been exposed to early adversity may possess an adequate reserve of 'protective' cognitions, such as optimistic biases and other beliefs that exempt them from the role of being a victim. Research has demonstrated that life events having salience to negative cognitive biases tend to have a depressogenic impact (Parker et al., 2000).

A common example of a 'key and lock' sequence would be somebody who was extensively criticised by a parent for being (say) 'stupid'. In later life, a colleague or intimate might malignantly or innocently state that that person had done something 'stupid', and thereby precipitate a disproportionately severe depressive response. Our argument is that the particular word is painfully evocative and salient as it mirrors earlier trauma and distressing circumstances. Sometimes such sequences are less straightforward. For instance, one woman developed a particularly marked depressive disorder following open-heart surgery. Pursuing the meaning of the surgery to her, she used words such as 'invaded' and 'violated', somewhat unusual words to use in that context. As she talked on, she described having been sexually assaulted when a young girl. Given an explanation she was reasonably prompt in making connections, recognising that when certain events occurred against her will she would be at particular risk of developing a depressive response. In other less fortunate cases, however, the simple recollection of a previous traumatic event may not necessarily alleviate current distress and other 'keys', such as pervasive cognitive schemas, may have to be sought.

In our research studies (Parker et al., 1998b; Parker et al., 2000), we quantified the relevance of the 'key and lock' model to differing depressive sub-types. The prevalence was highest for those with a clinical diagnosis of 'reactive depression', again supporting the revisionist view that formal categories such as 'reactive depression' or 'adjustment disorder with depressed mood' more reflect a state induced by the salience of the life event rather than by its severity.

As noted earlier, life events per se are less relevant than life events as perceived by the individual, in terms of their capacity to induce depression. Thus, many 'attribution theories' have been promulgated seeking to explain the influence of the experiential world (as against the 'real world') on depression. Some researchers have suggested that depression may arise when an individual's value system is compromised by external events or by conflict with another system of values. Throughout life, we evaluate good from bad, normal from abnormal, right from wrong, the acceptable from the unacceptable, and the important from the trivial. We make judgements in order to organise and give meaning to the world around us. If upheld rigidly, an individual's set of values may create vulnerability to depression when those values are challenged. Rigid attributional and perceptual styles can also serve as risk factors to depression. Attributional style is the global way in which individuals explain the cause of life events to themselves. For example, it incorporates the recognition of whether the cause and outcome of adverse events are within the control of the individual, whether such events are temporary or permanent, and whether such events affect one area of lifestyle or several. Perceptual style incorporates the ability (or lack thereof) to critically examine adverse experiences realistically in terms of their magnitude, locus of control, and helplessness and hopelessness for the future.

Nevertheless, it is important to bear in mind that not all salient stressors induce depressive episodes. Some stressors may in fact promote resilience, a construct that will be discussed in greater detail in Chapter 11. Resilience to future stressors occurs when an individual is allowed to develop valuable coping (behavioural and cognitive) strategies to current stressors. Attributional and perceptual styles may also be challenged by stressful events. If an individual is flexible enough to adopt a new set of attributions and perceptual biases taking into account current contingencies, then we may consider them to be resilient. However, if they cannot shift their rigid attributional and perceptual styles despite evidence to the contrary, they may be vulnerable to depressive episodes. Sometimes such increased resilience requires having gone 'through the fire' in order to re-work values, responses, and coping repertoires. In managing non-melancholic depression, the clinician needs to determine the strategies that could be successfully employed to improve resilience, a topic that will be discussed in Chapter 11.

11

Resilience and vulnerability in non-melancholic depression

In Chapters 8–10, we defined three components to the development of a non-melancholic disorder. Our emphasis in these chapters was on disorder risk, vulnerability, and their contribution to disorder onset. This is helpful to understand how an individual may become depressed and how treatment might assist. It is also important to consider the opposing pole of resilience, for strategies need to be applied to assist people to stay well and not experience repeated episodes. Thus, we now consider 'Resilience'.

In her book entitled 'Resilience', Deveson (2003) observes that, although the concept is difficult to define, we all seem to know it and we can usually identify those whom we would call 'resilient'. In the Oxford English Dictionary, resiliency is referred to as the ability to rebound or resume shape after stretching, not dissimilar to Hooke's Law. When used in the context of psychological well-being, resiliency usually refers to the recuperative power of an individual in coping with extreme or unusual stressors, such as a serious financial loss or the breakup of an important relationship. Definitions of resilience and resiliency have also changed over time to reflect some of the key virtues of a given society at a certain time. For example, 300 years ago, the ability of black slaves in America to tolerate and survive their numerous hardships would not have been regarded as particularly noteworthy. Yet today, their survival and adaptation within a hostile society is regarded as a testimony to their resilience.

There is tentative evidence to suggest that resilience may be more than simply the ability to 'bounce back' to a previous level of functioning following adversity. There are several examples in the popular press and in historical biographies of resilient people being fundamentally altered in some way following a severe life event. For example, the newspapers have often related stories of natural disaster survivors who have changed their life goals or devoted their life to helping others in similar circumstances. In this way, the term may also be used in the context of positive growth, adaptation, and change that leave an individual emotionally stronger and ultimately empower-ed to handle future stressors. Other definitions of resilience include:

1. The ability to withstand multiple and chronic stressors, and not lose one's sense of purpose.
2. Being able to draw on inner strengths to keep going in the face of adversity.
3. The ability to demonstrate persistence and fortitude in continuing on in one's chosen path, despite setbacks.
4. The ability to confront adversity but retain hope and meaning in life.
5. The ability to grow or to find new meanings in adversity.
6. Being able to hope for and believe in the possibility of a better life.

Vulnerability to depressive episodes

Some people are vulnerable to developing a depressive episode at some point in their lifetime. Such vulnerabilities may include genetic predisposition including a family history of depressive disorders, temperament and person-ality styles, history of childhood adversity, or current overwhelming life stres-sors. Specific types of vulnerabilities play a greater role in the onset of some depressive disorders. For example, in melancholic depression, biochemical changes or metabolic imbalances contribute to a greater extent to the onset of the illness than temperament and personality styles. The reverse is true for non-melancholic depression. In the latter case, such vulnerabilities may include heightened reactivity to stress, poor coping styles, ineffective problem-solving skills, interpersonal communication difficulties, and dysfunctional cognitive schemas. Little is known about those who are resilient to develop-ing depressive disorders but we can speculate that they do not have a genetic predisposition or a family history of these disorders and have not been exposed to extreme childhood adversity. Furthermore, they may have also developed effective skills at problem-solving, arousal modulation, interper-sonal communication and other coping repertoires, thus lessening the like-lihood that they would be exposed to or undermined by stressful life events.

Another type of vulnerability is that related to suffering from recurrent episodes of depression. The World Health Organization has documented the recurrent nature of depressive disorders in reporting that, following a single episode, the likelihood of another episode is 50%. After two episodes, the chances of suffering another episode increases to 70% and after three episodes, this figure increases to 90%. These figures are startling as one would expect that, with each episode of depression, individuals would become better at detecting early warning signs and in applying strategies that would prevent the onset of depression. Instead, the reverse happens and we see an increased likelihood of further depressive episodes.

Why, after just a single episode of depression, does one become more susceptible to further episodes of depression? One possibility is that neurochemical pathways in the brain become sensitised to minute perturbations which then trigger off another depressive disorder. But how does this occur? Why do not these minor perturbations just rectify themselves with time? How do these small changes in brain neurochemistry result in the neurotransmitter problems associated with the onset of an episode of depression. While there are likely to be multiple explanations depending on the type of depressive disorder, let us consider one possibility that may be especially relevant to non-melancholic depression:

1. Minute changes in brain chemistry could occur as a result of physical stressors such as lack of sleep (sleep deprivation), dietary effects such as getting drunk (alcohol intoxication), or metabolic changes, some of which may be inherited. Such changes could also occur when we watch a sad movie, a friend tells us of a distressing event, or we think about something sad.

2. Physical sensations (such as feeling tired or teary), which may be associated with these changes in brain chemistry, may trigger a number of unpleasant cognitive schemas or distressing memories. Most of these cognitive schemas and memories occur out of our awareness. Individuals may just find themselves interpreting their day-to-day activities in a particularly negative way or daydreaming about unpleasant events.

3. This process, unless interrupted, could then lead to further changes in brain neurochemistry which herald the early stages of a depressed mood. A depressed mood could then trigger further negative appraisals of events and the possibility of dwelling on other unpleasant memories, exacerbating neurotransmitter problems. In some, this vicious downward spiral will result in another depressive episode.

This tentative explanation lends itself to developing a model of building resilience based on focusing on developing strengths rather than solely on eliminating risk factors. Such an approach is consistent with that espoused in narrative therapy which helps people draw on their previous experiences of success in order to overcome their current difficulties. This model will be further developed in Chapters 12 and 13, which focus on intervention strategies for non-melancholic depression.

Resilience to further episodes of depression

As mentioned earlier, some individuals have not suffered from a depressive illness while others, after a single episode, do not suffer from further episodes of depression. We refer to these people as 'resilient'. But what sets them apart from others who are not so fortunate?

Resilience to developing a depressive illness is often a product of several factors, including positive self-regard and self-esteem, a sense of self-efficacy, good problem-solving skills, and the ability to manage and maintain anxiety at an adaptive level. It also usually reflects the culmination of a number of adaptive strategies which, used repeatedly, have served to prevent the development of long-standing lifestyle problems which may exacerbate the effects of other unexpected and uncontrollable stressors. People who are resilient to developing a depressive disorder may still become extremely distressed when confronted by certain types of stressors. However, they are able to move beyond the adverse experience and utilise strategies such as problem-solving or self-soothing techniques in order to ameliorate the stressor itself or modulate their response to it.

Components of resilience to depressive disorders include:

- positive self-image,
- high self-esteem and self-confidence,
- sense of self-efficacy,
- effective problem-resolution skills,
- arousal-modulation skills.

People vary in their levels of personal resilience to depressive disorders and differ in their reactions to different types of stressors. Some may be particularly resilient to economic hardship yet exquisitely sensitive to interpersonal conflict. Others may be able to weather the difficulties associated with a protracted legal dispute yet crumble at the notion of having to look after a sick child. The concept of vulnerability is closely entwined with that of resilience and may, to some extent, be regarded as its mirror opposite. Vulnerability to depression can result when a series of specific 'risk factors' co-occur to create serious problems in living skills or highly dysfunctional lifestyles that impact on self-esteem. Repeated episodes of depression can increase risk of further vulnerabilities through, among other things, lowering self-esteem, and encouraging a sense of poor mastery or limited self-efficacy, and negative self-image.

Increasing resilience to depression

In children, resilience to depression may be increased by the provision of an early childhood environment that is secure and comforting whist being both stimulating and supportive. Such an environment is thought to help establish the foundations of good self-esteem and confidence. In adults, resilience may be promoted by:

1. establishing connections with the people around us;
2. developing a sense of purpose in one's life;

3. having strong religious beliefs or a sense of spirituality;
4. changing the way we engage with and respond to life events;
5. 'isolating' or quarantining stressors so that they are separate to the sense of self;
6. deconstructing stressors and handling each smaller stress separately;
7. developing a sense of community or working for the common good;
8. having a sense of connection with a previous time of life, which offers respite from stress;
9. developing a framework for mastery over the environment;
10. making sense of events and making sense of the stressors we encounter.

Maintaining flexibility and adaptability

While the suggestions discussed earlier are thought to promote resilience, none is likely to be equally effective for all people all of the time. Often, we have to maintain a degree of flexibility in choosing how we address particular life events that have the potential to bring on a depressive episode and modify our response to suit the nature of the problem. While some problems can eventually be solved, some problems cannot and may require skills that help us to 'disengage' from them, a technique advocated in mindfulness therapy (Segal et al., 2002).

Using our model of vulnerability, we suggest that those that are resilient to further depressive episodes may have learnt how to distance themselves from transient unpleasant mood states rather than dwelling on them and eventually spiralling downwards into a full-blown depressive episode. For example, a resilient individual may note that they are not feeling quite themselves one day – perhaps they had a very late night or a busy week. They may be more likely to dismiss any negative thoughts and associated cognitive schemas as simply a function of their current state of mind which is due to sleep deprivation or physical and mental exhaustion. Thus, rather than spiralling into a depressive episode, they may acknowledge to themselves that they feel 'seedy' or 'down' but then continue unimpeded with their usual day-to-day activities.

In this instance, actively searching for strategies to lift one's mood may in fact cause more stress or distract from completing tasks. Sometimes it is better to just get on with day-to-day activities than to seek explanations or solutions to a mildly unpleasant mood. However, this is not the same as simply distracting one's attention from an unpleasant mood state. The key to resilience may be not only the willingness to acknowledge and accept a particularly unpleasant mood but to treat that mood state and its accompanying physical and psychological symptoms as external to one's sense of self and purpose.

Summary

Psychological intervention for depression aims to reduce distress in the short term and increase resilience in the long term. Many different types of therapies utilise some of the strategies listed above. In our later treatment chapters, a number of interventions will be detailed but here we conclude with a special point. Many therapies are designed to focus on an individual's vulnerabilities and limitations, appropriate and understandable. But people also benefit from having their strengths and positive attributes defined and harnessed in their treatment plans.

12

Psychological interventions for non-melancholic depression

We argue that the treatment of depressive disorders should reject the 'one size fits all' model in favour of a model based on a matrix of differing depressive disorders and a more differentiated 'horses for courses' management model of treatment. The three-tiered Black Dog Institute hierarchical model for depressive classes lends itself to the development of specific targeted interventions that can be expected to lead to higher rates of treatment efficacy. Further refinements in improving treatment efficacy are also possible by varying the levels or stages of intervention within each of the depressive classes. Varying the type and level of intervention enables treatment to be delivered at a more or less intensive level depending on symptom severity, chronicity, and complexity or comorbidity with other disorders.

The match between patients' and therapists' expectations is crucial for therapy to proceed effectively. A mismatch, unless resolved, becomes a source of distraction and irritation in therapy. Although, if designed by an experienced therapist, such a mismatch can be used to advantage to shift patients' rigid expectations and may be especially useful in treating those with highly dysfunctional personality styles.

Psychological interventions for non-melancholic depression

Recent studies on the treatment of depressive disorders have predominantly focused on pharmacological or other biological therapies, most notably the efficacy of antidepressant medications. Explanations of the origins of depressive symptoms have focused on describing and categorising the various neurotransmitter pathways in the brain that may be responsible for particular physical and/or psychological phenomena. Though these studies are highly valuable in terms of increasing our understanding of 'depression', by and large they do not explain the complex interplay between (among other things) premorbid personality factors, maladaptive behavioural repertoires, and acute and/or chronic life stressors, especially in the treatment and management of non-melancholic depressions.

Psychological formulations of non-melancholic depression can often offer credible and clinically useful explanations for most depressive symptoms, as well as plausible explanations for the onset, course, and maintenance of depressive episodes. Interventions based on these formulations can offer patients a degree of control over their illness by allowing them to actively participate in the treatment process.

There are many different forms of psychological interventions, with all claiming to be effective in treating depression. As noted, differences in therapeutic efficacy between various psychological treatments which claim to work in different ways appears to be minimal, posing the question as to whether all therapies are as effective as each other. Furthermore, the overwhelming popularity of alternative or natural therapies and the success of self-help books attest to the fact that many people suffering from depression select therapies based on their own opinions of what may be helpful to them. Treatment choices may be based on several factors including level of media coverage for a specific form of treatment, advice from significant others, and cost and convenience, among other things.

Although there are many studies examining the efficacy of the various psychological treatments, there is a dearth of empirical information about the active ingredients of each of these therapies and their mechanisms of action. Each intervention emphasises different aspects of the therapeutic process as the main ingredient for change. Some may emphasise awareness of repressed conflicts and the attainment of insight, while others may stress the importance of the therapeutic relationship, and still others may focus on behavioural and/or cognitive change. The way in which therapists choose a particular orientation is also an intriguing question in its own right and may reflect their training, personality style or their impressions of what may be beneficial to their clients. There are also many therapists who claim to work within an eclectic framework, adopting a flexible approach that allows them to adapt to the needs of their patients rather than having the patient adapt to the therapist's particular therapeutic approach.

Active ingredients common to any psychological intervention are thought to include:
1. patient characteristics,
2. therapist characteristics,
3. therapy characteristics, and
4. interactive effects between all these components.

Patient characteristics

In the non-melancholic depressions, we argue that temperament and personality factors play a key role in the development, maintenance, and course of recovery from an episode of depression. These characteristics can shape the surface symptom pattern and determine, to some extent, the likelihood of treatment compliance and the probability of relapse.

Other patient characteristics include a history of prior treatment failures which can affect motivation to seek treatment and adherence to a treatment program. The level of social support, long-standing marital discord or psychosocial adversity can also affect response to psychological interventions.

Therapist characteristics

Several therapist characteristics are thought to influence the course and outcome of therapy independently of therapy type. Warmth, empathy and genuineness or sincerity are thought to be very important. Spontaneity and humour are also considered to be important ingredients which help to enliven the process of psychological treatment.

A depressed patient may not be capable of generating the level of enthusiasm required to actively participate in the therapeutic process in the early stages of therapy. Genuine optimism, hope, and encouragement by the therapist about the outcome of therapy are of special relevance to patients suffering from a depressive disorder. Another therapist characteristic is an openness to discuss issues concerning the therapeutic process itself. Patients who have been allowed to ventilate their frustrations, grievances, or concerns about current and past efforts at therapy, and who feel that their views are respected by their therapist, are more likely to adhere to and comply with treatment.

Therapy characteristics

Convenience of the therapy in terms of location, timing, and duration are important therapy characteristics that can influence outcome and adherence to treatment. Level of discomfort associated with the treatment itself or with side effects, the provision of an adequate rationale for the treatment process, and whether the treatment is acceptable to the patient's cultural, social, financial, and educational background are also important characteristics of appropriate psychological intervention.

Therapies that help operationalise the signs and symptoms of depression at various times throughout treatment may help patients develop treatment goals and provide a benchmark for improvement over time. As many depressed patients have difficulty in focusing on specific problems, therapies that help operationalise problems may be more helpful than 'undirected' therapies.

Some therapies encourage the involvement of a spouse or other significant people to provide support and encouragement to the patient and help re-establish and re-engage the patient within their social and family networks during the course of therapy. The process of involving others may include psycho-education about the patient's condition, progress, and outcome of therapy.

Interactive effects

The establishment of a good therapeutic alliance is a feature common to most, if not all, therapeutic approaches to treating depression. The ability to include the patient in the collaborative nature of the treatment appears to be an important therapy ingredient. Setting reasonable expectations regarding the duration and likely benefit of therapy should be part of a comprehensive assessment of the patient. The assessment should also establish a shared context for therapy and problem formulation (i.e. the causes or precipitants, vulnerability, exacerbatory and maintenance factors, and goals for therapy). Also critical to the success of therapy is the transmission of the belief that change is possible and an expectancy that the depression will eventually lift.

Psychological therapies for non-melancholic depression

Cognitive and behavioural therapies

Cognitive-based therapies address dysfunctional cognitive schemas and specific dysfunctional cognitions associated with the current depressive episode (Beck et al., 1979; McCullough Jr., 2000; Parker, 2002). Negative schemas are global negative thoughts about the way in which events in the world are perceived and judged ('cognitive errors'). Dysfunctional cognitions associated with depression are thought to form a negative 'cognitive triad' comprising negative views about the self, current life experiences, and the future. Dysfunctional cognitions associated with the current depressive episode are usually more amenable to change than the more entrenched cognitive schemas. Therapies aimed at changing dysfunctional thoughts aim to help sufferers identify, challenge, and change these cognitive patterns.

Behavioural strategies are usually aimed at bringing the patient's behaviours back to their previous levels before the current depressive episode began. One theory for the onset of some depressive disorders is based on the 'learned helplessness' model of Martin Seligman (1975). 'Learned helplessness' is thought to result when an individual learns that he cannot control those elements of his life that may relieve suffering, bring gratification, or provide nurturance. If a patient believes that he is helpless to change or control aversive life events, he will develop an episode of depression. In treatment, forced exposure to making appropriate or adaptive responses to gain rewards can help to alleviate depression by restoring a sense of self-efficacy. The model also suggests that learned helplessness can be prevented if an individual has prior exposure to mastery over major life events.

Combining the two types of strategies has resulted in the development of a number of cognitive behavioural therapies which help patients identify, reality–test and correct distorted conceptualisations and dysfunctional beliefs (schemas). Cognitive behavioural therapies aim to:

(i)   teach patients to identify and monitor negative, dysfunctional, and distressing thoughts that are automatically triggered by certain events;

(ii) recognise the causative connections between thoughts, feelings, and behaviours;

(iii) examine the evidence for and against distorted or dysfunctional thoughts;

(iv) substitute more reality-oriented interpretations for biased interpretations of events;

(v)   learn to identify and alter those dysfunctional beliefs which predispose towards distorted experiences.

Cognitive behavioural therapies also offer patients 'hope', control, and mastery, ongoing contact with a professional therapist and help to make sense of their personal world. These types of therapies also provide patients with a credible plan for recovery including a rationale for therapy. They offer a high degree of structure with logical sequences and achievable goals, training in the independent use of effective skills, as well as demonstrating that it is possible to change attributions for events, and to develop a sense of self-efficacy and mastery over events in their immediate environments.

Interpersonal psychotherapy

Interpersonal psychotherapy (IPT) targets specific areas of 'deficit' in the interpersonal domain and aims to resolve unpleasant changes in the patient's social network that may be caused by and/or perpetuate the depressive episode (Klerman & Weissman, 1994; Stuart & Robertson, 2003). The general goal of IPT is to improve the social adjustment of the patient and thereby alleviate symptoms of depression. Successfully treated patients are thus able to solve their own interpersonal problems and pursue their own life goals, free of the disorder that brought them to therapy. IPT outcome goals are linked to the four interpersonal areas of 'grief', 'interpersonal conflict', 'role transition', and 'interpersonal deficit'. Only one interpersonal area is usually selected by mutual agreement between the patient and therapist as the focus for intervention during the first few sessions.

Specific goals of therapy may vary according to the interpersonal domain selected. For example, if the interpersonal area selected is grief, then the goals of therapy are:

1. to facilitate the mourning process associated with loss, and
2. to assist the individual to form new and rewarding relationships.

If the interpersonal area is that of interpersonal conflict, then the goals for treatment may be:

1. to identify the nature of the interpersonal conflict,
2. decide on a plan of remedial action, and
3. implement the action plan, including strategies such as improving communication skills or teaching skills in conflict resolution.

If role transition is the problem area, then the goals of treatment would be to:

1. facilitate mourning and acceptance of the loss of an old role,
2. help the patient regard their new role in a positive framework, and
3. restore their self-esteem and confidence by progressive mastery of the demands of the new role.

For patients who present with interpersonal deficits, the goals would be:

1. to reduce social isolation, and
2. assist them in establishing new and rewarding relationships.

Narrative therapy

Narrative therapy is about listening to how patients relate their problems as life 'stories' (Epstein & White, 1992). By attempting to understand patients' stories, the therapist develops trust and rapport with the patient. In addition, the therapist gains ideas about how those stories may restrict patients from overcoming their difficulties. Therapists are instructed to actively listen to patients' stories without reifying undesirable meanings. This technique is referred to as 'deconstructive listening' and is usually accomplished by clarifying the meanings of stories and asking 'what if ...?' or 'could it be that …?' questions. Other techniques used in narrative therapy include:

- 'deconstructive questioning' or re-examining stories from a different perspective,
- listening and asking about possible alternate stories,
- helping patients develop new stories,
- questioning patients on how they arrived at a particular conclusion,
- asking for more detail in order to get patients to analyse the logic embedded within their stories,
- asking for the 'meaning' of particular points in the stories,
- extending the stories in time and examining the putative consequences.

The overall aim of Narrative Therapy is to make life events 'significant' for the patient by examining how they might learn from their previous life experiences and apply similar strategies, particularly when they had coped successfully. Sometimes individuals are also encouraged to document their thoughts about events and their impact on them in terms of problem resolution and their future life. They may also be asked to consider how their behaviours may hinder them from achieving what they really want in life.

Solution-focused therapies

Therapies grouped under this heading are those that heavily focus on short-term, 'task-oriented', adaptive solutions to problems (Furman & Ahola, 1994). The purpose of these forms of brief therapy is not necessarily to 'understand' the cause of a given problem, but rather to find novel ways of conceptualising the problem together with practical solutions for dealing with it. As the emphasis of therapy is on solutions, therapists may encourage patients to discuss problems and other issues in a manner that tends to generate and encourage optimism, collaboration, and trust in the patient's own resources.

Solution-focused therapies aim to provide pleasant experiences that turn problems into challenges, foster optimism, enhance collaboration, inspire creativity, and help clients retain their dignity. They usually comprise three parts which:

1. address different levels of patient motivation,
2. help patients maintain the changes they make in treatment, and
3. prevent the recurrence of the problem.

Specific solution-focused techniques include:

- inventing creative names and labels for problems,
- making up alternate explanations for problems,
- viewing the past as a 'positive' experience,

- recognising and acknowledging the patient's expertise in overcoming their problems,
- sharing personal experiences with the therapist,
- generating creative solutions, and
- creating positive future visions.

Psychotherapies

The term 'psychotherapy' encompasses a number of therapies originally developed from psychoanalytic techniques that were predominantly based on the work of Sigmund Freud. While earlier versions of formal psychodynamic psychotherapy extended over lengthy periods of time and with frequent sessions (sometimes several times a week and for several years), more recent types of psychotherapies, such as 'brief' psychodynamic psychotherapy, are of shorter duration and with clearer treatment goals. Most psychotherapies utilise, to some extent, the patient–client relationship in order to understand how the patient acts in everyday life and to effect change, for example, focusing on the emotions generated during the therapy sessions towards the therapist or on resistance to change. In the treatment of depression, such therapies may also focus on how the individual developed their current episode of depression, or on early childhood issues (such as harsh, punitive parenting, or childhood abuse) that have led to a propensity to develop depressive episodes. While the main aim of brief psychotherapy is to assist in the development of insight, the support and encouragement offered by such therapy ('supportive psychotherapy') can also greatly benefit depressed individuals.

The effectiveness of psychotherapy depends, to a large extent, on the skills of the therapist and the readiness and ability of the patient to embark on the process of therapy. Although it can be especially helpful for some with non-melancholic depression, it is not recommended as a primary treatment for psychotic or melancholic depression.

Counselling

Like psychotherapy, counselling covers a range of therapy styles which generally focus on crisis intervention and problem-solving. The role of the therapist is to help the patient clarify and prioritise key problem areas, identify those that need to be addressed, and encourage and support patients to act on their problems, and review their progress. There are several specialities within the realm of counselling including marital counselling and career or vocational advice. Crisis counselling not only involves problem-solving skills but may also include elements of stress- and anxiety-management techniques.

Problem-solving skills

Although regarded as a specific type of intervention rather than a therapy modality in its own right, the provision and enhancement of problem-solving skills is such an effective intervention that it warrants a special place in this section. Promoting problem-solving skills enable depressed individuals to focus their attentions and energies on productive activities which will ultimately reduce their level of stress and improve their situation. Although there are many different types of problem-solving strategies, a simple and popular technique is outlined as follows:

1. Describe and define the problem as clearly as possible,
2. Consider several solutions (without censure) to the problem, being as creative as possible,
3. Examine each solution for its advantages and disadvantages,
4. Decide on a single solution or a combination of several solutions which can be implemented simultaneously or sequentially,
5. Implement the solution(s),
6. Review progress over a reasonable period of time, and
7. Refine solution(s) or try another solution if unsuccessful.

Problem-solving techniques are usually used in combination with other types of therapies as an effective way to minimise or eliminate ongoing stressors that could be exacerbating a depressive episode, particularly for the non-melancholic disorders.

Other types of therapies

There are many other therapies that we have not addressed in this chapter. This omission is not intended to imply that they are any less effective than the ones described here. Rather, we have described some of the more commonly used and better-researched therapies that are accessible to a wide range of mental health professionals.

Intervention strategies for non-melancholic depression

Rather than attempting to fit a particular type of therapy to each of the personality styles that are relevant to the development of non-melancholic depression, we have chosen to adopt a more targeted approach to treatment.

Thus, in the ensuing chapters we shall weave in components from these and other types of therapies to address the issues relevant to the different personality styles in non-melancholic depression. Rather than encourage therapists to provide a particular type of therapy non-specifically (where the patient is 'fitted' to a particular therapy), we argue for a reverse process of fitting and melding therapeutic components to the individual's points of vulnerability: a pluralistic model.

In Chapter 13 we consider, in some detail, how the stress-related and personality-weighted non-melancholic disorders can be assisted by pluralistic clinical strategies.

Part IV

Modelling and managing the non-melancholic depressive disorders

In Chapters 12–22, we detail the separate contribution of life stress-determined as well as personality-determined non-melancholic depressive disorders as if they are separate 'types'. In reality, and as detailed earlier in the book, they are interdependent rather than independent, so that any one individual is likely to have their non-melancholic disorder determined by a mix of contributory personality styles and variable life event stressor patterns.

While recognising this complexity, we nevertheless consider each contributor in a separate chapter, with the view that this approach allows each stressor, response and personality style to be considered by itself and with attendant advantages. In clinical practice, the clinician needs to consider such interdependencies in formulating a pluralistic treatment plan, to ensure that component parts (as considered here) are modelled to explain and manage the whole pattern.

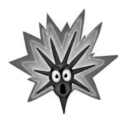

13

Acute stress-related non-melancholic depression

A depressive disorder commonly develops following a recent severe stressful event. When the stressor is severe and/or salient and seemingly explanatory of the depressive 'response', the depressive episode is commonly labelled 'acute' or 'reactive' in nature. Two types of stressful events may precipitate such a response:

1. Those usually characterised by a significant degree of uncontrollability but not necessarily unpredictability, that are regarded as distressing to the vast majority of people (e.g. the breakup of a close relationship or severe financial loss). Individual responses to acute stressors such as these may verge on helplessness and inactivity. While this form of depression (Type 1 acute non-melancholic depression) has a high rate of 'spontaneous' recovery in the short term, for some it may persist for several months and lead to secondary problems, thereby worsening the depressive episode.

2. Those that, while seeming to be relatively insignificant, may precipitate a depressive reaction that is out of proportion to the magnitude of the event itself (e.g. over-reacting and getting extremely upset in response to minor criticism from a friend). A 'key and lock' model best describes this sequence and the reactions generated, and which we refer to as Type 2 acute non-melancholic depression.

These two expressions of acute non-melancholic depression are described in the two following chapters. Treatment implications are based on a model of 'stepped care' where a number of strategic techniques are employed as a first level of intervention (described in this chapter) and a second level of more intensive interventions (described in Chapter 14) may be used if necessary.

The psychotransmitter model

We can use an 'agonist model' as an analogy to describe the development of an episode of non-melancholic depression in response to an acute

Fig. 13.1 Stressor
saliency and flood of
psychotransmitter.

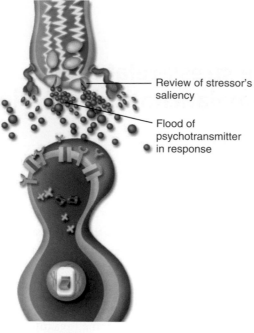

Review of stressor's
saliency

Flood of
psychotransmitter
in response

Fig. 13.2
Psychotransmitter
bombardment.

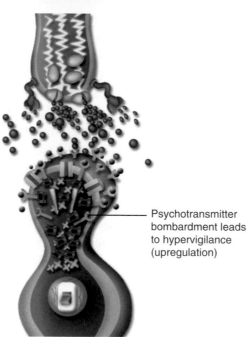

Psychotransmitter
bombardment leads
to hypervigilance
(upregulation)

major life event. In this model, a powerful and salient stimulus (life event)
generates an overload of a depressogenic psychotransmitter which floods
across the synapse to bombard the post-synaptic neuron. In response to
this overload, the receiving neuron first begins creating new receptors (akin

Fig. 13.3
Hyperarousal results
in receptor
destruction.

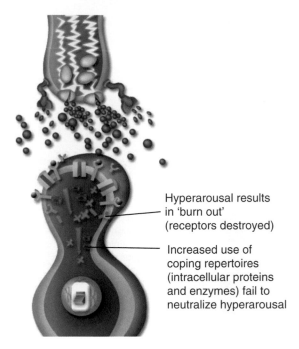

Hyperarousal results
in 'burn out'
(receptors destroyed)

Increased use of
coping repertoires
(intracellular proteins
and enzymes) fail to
neutralize hyperarousal

to concentrating and attending to the stressor). This process is referred to as 'upregulation', resulting in increased receptor density (here, focusing on the stressor) in accordance with high concentrations of psychotransmitter molecules in the synapse (Figs 13.1 and 13.2).

As the psychotransmitter bombardment continues, the post-synaptic neuron becomes overwhelmed and exhausted as 'intracellular' activity level increases. Depletion of energy (anergia and fatigue) occurs, as the neuron has to quickly remove and destroy receptors (akin to 'ignoring' the aversive stressor as well as other forms of stimulation including more pleasurable ones) from the cell membrane to halt the level of activity ('down-regulation'). The abrupt slowing down of cellular activity and the creation of second messengers which reflect a depleted sense of mastery has a rapid cascade effect 'shutting down' self-esteem ('giving up response') and causing depression (Figs 13.3 and 13.4).

This model relies on the interplay of:
- A flood of psychotransmitters.
- Receptor overload.
- Cellular up-regulation and then down-regulation compromising altered coping functioning.
- Processes that eventually shut down self-esteem.

Fig. 13.4 Depletion of sense of mastery and 'shutting down' self-esteem.

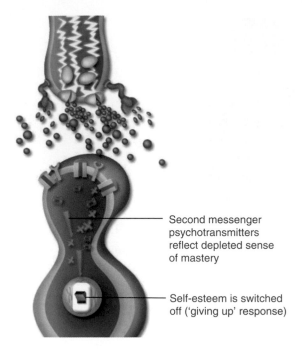

Second messenger psychotransmitters reflect depleted sense of mastery

Self-esteem is switched off ('giving up' response)

Treatment strategies in this instance would involve removing or neutralising the stimulus (life event), a process which would immediately, or over time, help restore the optimal level of receptor concentration and allow intracellular proteins (coping strategies) to facilitate the turning on of self-esteem.

Case vignette – Dave

Dave is a 47-year-old married father of three school-aged children who had been retrenched from his work 2 months ago. Although he understood the reasons for his retrenchment, he nevertheless became increasingly depressed as his attempts to find work met with failure and disappointment. He began to worry about several aspects of his life including his future, the likelihood of ever finding suitable employment and his ongoing financial commitments. He was especially concerned about discussing his retrenchment with his friends at the local club. Over the previous few weeks, Dave's sleep was disturbed, he had lost his appetite, and was constantly tired. His wife, though very supportive at first, was beginning to tire of Dave's depressed mood and pessimistic outbursts. At first, she had tried to cheer him up by reassuring him that he would eventually find work and that this was an opportunity for him to spend more time with her and the children. But as the weeks dragged on, Dave's mood and pessimism worsened, and neither she nor the children enjoyed spending time with him.

Case summary

Dave's depressive episode was precipitated by the loss of his job in a company he had been working in for several years. Apart from the economic stressors, Dave had also lost his status as a provider for his family and as a company executive among his friends. The stress of losing his job may have touched on a number of issues underpinning his self-esteem and self-confidence. In addition, the burden of financial insecurity and possible future hardship through the loss of his job had put considerable strain on his relationship with his wife and children. As he attempted to 'cope harder' (e.g. redoubling his efforts to find a new job) and such coping failed, he felt more demoralised and then exhausted.

Summary of Dave's problem areas

- Feelings of loss of status among his family and friends.
- Loss of self-esteem and sense of self-efficacy.
- Anxiety about possible financial hardship and employment insecurity.
- Feelings of helplessness.
- Strain on family relationships.

Principles of psychological intervention

Brief time-limited therapy with clearly stated realistic goals and with a strong focus on problem-solving strategies should be useful in this type of depressive presentation. It is essential that psychological intervention proceeds at a rapid pace; for example by scheduling frequent but short sessions with clear behavioural goals. Problem-solving strategies could be used to ameliorate specific aspects of the current stressor and can reap secondary gain in improving self-esteem and self-confidence. Other strategies, such as advice and constructive suggestions by the therapist, can also be useful in lessening the impact of current stressors. Other important therapy characteristics include the development of a collaborative plan for intervention, the provision of relevant information, and monitoring ongoing progress.

A structure for psychological intervention
- Brief time-limited therapy.
- Clearly stated realistic goals.
- Strong focus on problem-solving strategies.

- Improve self-esteem and self-confidence.
- Advice and constructive suggestions by the therapist.
- Collaborative intervention plan.
- Provision of relevant information.
- Monitoring ongoing progress.

What sort of therapist?

A therapeutic alliance based on mutual collaboration around problem-solving will be crucial to the success of psychological intervention. The therapist could mention his or her own experience in helping others in similar circumstances. Discussion of some of the common methods used in overcoming similar types of adversities can help to create a sense of collaboration with the patient and promote hope for the future.

Getting started

People suffering from an episode of depression precipitated by an acute stressor will frequently seek treatment from their general practitioner initially. Somatic complaints such as sleep difficulties, muscle aches and pains, or headaches are among the most common symptoms (in addition to depression) reported by these individuals. A first step in any intervention is to educate the client that the physical ailments may in fact reflect a depressive episode brought about by stress. Information in the form of reading material, pamphlets or books on stress and depression will help to provide a rationale for psychological intervention.

Next, it is essential to determine and prioritise the specific areas for psychological and practical intervention. Problem areas could include financial difficulties such as meeting mortgage re-payments, conflicts with their partner who may feel overburdened, and feelings of loneliness or isolation from friends who are employed. Although all these areas may merit attention, an intervention plan would have to determine the relative importance of working on one area at the expense of another.

Establishing the areas for intervention

Identifying clear and achievable short-term goals for therapy is a priority before beginning any intervention programme. It is important to adhere to these goals as much as possible during the course of brief therapy despite the possibility of distraction by more immediate stressors. A useful technique is to document all the short-term goals. These can then be referred to throughout the course of psychological therapy.

Setting realistic goals

Establish short-term goals for therapy and make sure improvements can be assessed or measured at the end of treatment. For example:

Goals	Measurable goals
1. To feel better about self	To acknowledge successes however small (by keeping a diary of daily achievements)
2. To feel optimistic about the future	To stop entertaining pessimistic thoughts (by challenging negative thoughts)
3. To feel energised	To get involved in a program of regular exercise

---

Next, determine the main problem areas that need to be addressed over the course of therapy, based on the initial assessment.

Problem area	Psychological intervention
• Feeling of loss of status among family and friends	• Raising self-confidence and self-esteem; learning to acknowledge successes
• Anxiety about possible financial hardship and employment insecurity	• Anxiety-management skills
• Feelings of helplessness and ineffectiveness	• Problem-solving strategies
• Strain on family relationships	• Counselling and support for family

Intervention strategies

1. Raising self-confidence and self-esteem may be addressed by working on a number of behavioural tasks that have personal relevance and possibly influence the eventual resolution of the current stressor. For example, taking up a hobby, learning a new skill, or participating more fully in community activity can help boost self-confidence and self-esteem as well as increasing the likelihood of eventually finding a job.

2. Anxiety-management skills such as relaxation training, slow-breathing, and imaginal techniques are useful strategies for reducing high levels of autonomic arousal.

Relaxation training

While lying on a bed or sitting in a comfortable chair, focus on the large muscles in your body beginning with your feet (if you prefer, you may start with you face and work through those muscles first, slowly moving down through your body till you get to your feet). As you focus on each muscle group, imagine that any tension in these muscles is slowly draining away from your body, leaving those muscles in a state of complete relaxation. Work through all the parts of your body, such as your calf muscles, lower and upper back, shoulders, arms and hands, spending a little more time on any part that feels especially tense. When you get to your face, take the time to relax the muscles in your jaw, and around your eyes and forehead. When you finish working through all the muscle groups in your body, spend a few minutes just focusing on the feelings of complete relaxation. Practise this exercise twice a day, preferably once in the morning and again in the evening before you go to sleep.

Slow-breathing exercise

Sit in a chair and spend a couple of minutes focusing on your breathing. Once you feel that you can concentrate on your breathing, try to slow it down to the count of 3 seconds to breathe in and 3 seconds to breathe out. Do this for a few minutes and, after you achieve a rhythm, stop counting but say the word 'relax' to yourself as you breathe out. Practise this exercise two or three times a day and whenever you feel stressed.

Another useful technique to minimise worries and depressive ruminations is to simplify or 'contain' the issue of concern so it does not seem so daunting. This technique is called 'containing the problem' and is described below.

Containing the problem(s)

Imagine you could put all these problems into a large metal box with a padlock or a combination lock. Imagine placing them in there one-by-one. As you close the lid imagine that a mechanism in the box compresses all these problems into a small cube. You can open the box when you feel ready to face the small cube.
Or
Sit in a chair and imagine the problem(s) as a small fire at your feet. Close your eyes and imagine this fire as clearly as you can – the heat, the crackling sounds, and the smell. Imagine the fire beginning to burn itself out as it runs out of wood or paper until all you can see is a small pile of ashes.

3. Problem-solving techniques are especially useful in addressing individual stresses before they compound one another or become chronic. Identify a potential 'neutralising event' (NE) that would negate or neutralise the original stressor, and work towards achieving that end. For example, if the initial stressor was a job loss, then a potential NE would be to get the original job back or to get a new job. Either of these solutions would involve a range of problem-solving strategies depending on feasibility.

Problem-solving

Decide on a problem area and clarify the nature of the problem. For example, how would you ensure that the weekly grocery expenses do not exceed $200?

Apply possible solutions to that problem, such as shopping at the closest discount supermarket and taking only a limited amount of cash. Review success by deciding whether the budget was adequate for the week and whether modifications need to be made to the original solution.

4. Relationship counselling, perhaps in the form of education, joint problem-solving or scheduling weekly pleasant activities together may help restore emotional balance to strained partnerships. In some cases, family counselling may be necessary to ease family stressors.

Barriers to effective intervention

It is unlikely that long-term therapy is required in the treatment of an acute stress-related depressive episode. However, on occasion, without adequate resolution of the original stressor, this type of depression may develop into a more chronic type requiring additional intervention strategies. If this occurs, then it would be necessary to mutually negotiate a new intervention strategy with different short- and long-term goals.

The role of medication

The usefulness of medication varies from individual to individual with an acute stress-related non-melancholic depression. If an antidepressant is to be considered, then a selective serotonin reuptake inhibitor (SSRI) is clearly the first choice. For many individuals such drugs are helpful in muting the 'stress', modulating the high level of physiological arousal and lowering levels of worry. Other antidepressant classes are unlikely to be superior to SSRIs, and an alternative choice might be dictated by drug side-effect profiles. We would generally only commence antidepressant medication if (say over the first week) the patient had not shown a significant improvement following initial interview and assistance, and consider their role as adjunctive only.

Anxiolytic medication and sleeping tablets are often of assistance but, if prescribed, should only be for a brief period, as tolerance rapidly develops and the risks of addiction are high.

14

Acute stress-related non-melancholic depression: 'key and lock' model

A second type of expression of acute stress-driven non-melancholic depression is characterised by an intense emotional reaction that appears disproportionate to the stressor ('key and lock' model) which we refer to as Type 2. This stressor has particular salience to the depressed individual, often unlocking histories of previous emotionally charged or traumatic events. Individuals with expressions of Type 2 acute stress-related non-melancholic depression may not be immediately aware of the reasons for their intense reaction. Once these reasons are uncovered, usually with the help of a therapist, understanding and accepting the links with their past can help to alleviate many of their distressing symptoms and build resilience against future reactions of this type.

The psychotransmitter model

Some life events have particular salience for the development of non-melancholic depression. Using an agonist model once again, some types of depressogenic neurotransmitters (life events) with salient types of psychological configurations can rapidly dock and lock onto receptors (interpretation and reaction) and initiate high levels of cellular activity (stress). In response to that activity, channels open and remain opened (here, perceptual and attributIONal styles reinforce the interpretation of and reactions to life events), and continue to stimulate cellular activity to dangerous levels. The post-synaptic neuron once again becomes over-stimulated and has to expend energy in order to slow down cellular activity by removing receptors and thus closing the attributION channels which, in turn, also shuts down self-esteem (causing depression).

This model relies on the interplay of:
• Flood of psychotransmitters.

- Receptor hypersensitivity, reflecting developmental factors influencing selective neuronal wiring problems.
- Selective attributIONal channels being opened and then closed by the removal of receptors.
- Processes that directly shut down self-esteem.

In order to stop this reaction, one might prioritise decreasing receptor hypersensitivity (by identifying and addressing the salience of some life events) thus altering the mechanism whereby selective attributION channels are opened too readily (challenging and changing perceptual and attributional styles).

Case vignette – Karen

As a 5th-year medical student, Karen was beginning to contemplate whether or not to specialise when she completed her medical degree. During her practical term in surgery in a large teaching hospital, her supervisor, an irascible senior surgeon, yelled at her during a ward round about her inability to recall the name of a specific surgical procedure. Karen immediately became very depressed and quickly left the hospital booking herself into a motel where she planned her suicide. The experience had reminded her of her highly successful and overbearing businessman father who would often vociferously reprimand his children, especially Karen, in front of her other three siblings. Karen had always felt helpless to defend herself against her father's tirades and accusations which were often unfairly levelled at her. After one of her father's outbursts, Karen would become quiet, then withdraw to her bedroom where she would lie on her bed and cry tears of frustration over her powerlessness. Over the next few weeks following that ward round, Karen remained withdrawn and depressed over her perceived incompetence.

Case summary

Although Karen's depressive episode was precipitated by being publicly reprimanded by her medical supervisor, the incident itself (the 'key') mirrored previous similar incidents with her father in which she felt powerless and insecure (the 'lock'). Her current depressive episode was driven by the thoughts and emotions associated with the earlier and, at first pass, unrelated events in her past. Of particular relevance is the way in which specific aspects of the incident with her supervisor, such as his being a male authority figure possibly of the same generation as her father and exercising his displeasure at her performance, could elicit the same reactions that she felt at an earlier, and more vulnerable age.

Other 'key and lock' scenarios may be less obvious, and with the patient having no inkling about associations. For example, and as noted earlier, one woman after undergoing open-heart surgery, developed depression following a sense of being 'violated'. History taking identified early 'violations' (childhood sexual abuse) that had been long suppressed.

Summary of Karen's problem areas

- Lack of awareness regarding the depression trigger.
- Re-experience of thoughts and emotions associated with an earlier event.
- Feeling powerless and insecure.
- Feeling 'not good enough'.

Principles of psychological intervention

Short- to medium-term intervention is recommended for this type of depressive episode. Adopting a 'key and lock' approach to problem formulation and treatment requires exploration of previous incidents that may have elicited the same or similar sets of cognitions or emotions. The aim of psychological intervention would be to facilitate the development of insight into the reasons for current distress and to promote the recognition of possible triggers to future episodes. Once realised, a goal of psychological intervention would be to derive alternate ways of handling similar situations.

> **A structure for psychological intervention:**
> Short- to medium-term psychological intervention:
> - Focus on exploring previous situations which evoked the same or similar sets of cognitions and emotions.
> - Facilitate the development of insight in recognising the origins (the 'locks') of current distress.
> - Explore alternate ways of coping with such situations.

What sort of therapist?

A firm, trusting therapeutic relationship with a supportive therapist is important for recovery from this type of depression. Direct permission and encouragement to ventilate unpleasant emotions, such as frustration and anger, during the therapy sessions will be helpful. These emotions could be used to stimulate the recollection of previous situations which engendered the same or similar cognitions or reactions. The therapist would also need to be adept at facilitating the 'connection' between present and past incidents, using unpleasant emotional states as a common link.

Getting started

Recognition of the disproportionate nature of a persisting emotional reaction and its associated problems is usually what drives the need for treatment. Explanation of how a 'key and lock' model may be applicable to the situation can help reduce the level of distress, and provides a rationale for the joint exploration and uncovering of previous situations which elicited similar reactions. An important aspect of therapy is to draw on or highlight personal strengths and resilience in other, unrelated, situations. These strengths can then be used to refute dysfunctional cognitions, and poor self-confidence in the target situation.

Establishing the areas for intervention

A narrative approach to therapy would be advisable as a first step in this expression of non-melancholic depression. Using this approach, the therapist would encourage the patient to describe how current and previous problems may be inter-related and re-formulated as 'stories' linked by similar cognitions and emotional reactions. Each story would have a beginning, middle, and end point possibly extending into the future. Encouraging the patient to document these life stories and the meanings they extracted from those experiences could also provide insights into problem areas.

Other psychological techniques, such as anxiety-reduction strategies, could be introduced during the course of therapy to deal with specific areas of concern or problems with coping.

Problem area	Psychological intervention
• Lack of understanding regarding an emotional over-reaction to some events	• Use of questioning and interpretation by the therapist to guide personal reflection
• Negative emotional states that drive dysfunctional thinking styles	• Scheduling pleasant events and use of cognitive therapy to address negative thoughts
• Feelings of powerlessness regarding emotional reactions	• Identification of specific cues or triggers for adverse emotional reactions
• Heightened levels of arousal when upset	• Anxiety-reduction strategies

Intervention strategies

1. Questioning by the therapist of the circumstances surrounding the stressful event can often help to trigger memories of previous similar

events which link the present to the past. Such recollections can be distressing, especially if there are no established effective self-consolatory behaviours. It could be useful during the therapy sessions to document those events using a chart or timeline which also can illustrate periods of great strength or high resilience. Interpretation by the therapist of the reasons for high levels of distress can facilitate the process of self-reflection by the patient. If previous perturbing events are not readily identifiable, abreaction techniques, or hypnosis may be beneficial.

2. Deciding on, and scheduling pleasant events can help to lift mood and can also help to organise time otherwise spent in depressive ruminations. Pleasant activities need to be scheduled on a regular basis (e.g. daily), firstly with short activities of around 20 min. These activities can be extended to up to an hour per day.

Examples of pleasant activities:
- Taking a warm bath
- Sitting in the park
- Reading a favourite magazine
- Spending time with a pet
- Talking to a friend on the phone
- Enjoying a food treat.

It is necessary to challenge dysfunctional cognitions, especially those that feed issues of poor self-esteem and self-confidence. Using this approach, negative self-statements can be critically examined and challenged by using evidence of good coping skills or expertise in other unrelated situations. One technique is to focus on regular activity that is engaged in with reasonable and consistent success, such as cooking, fishing, or golfing. Then identify all the qualities that make such tasks successful. Next, examine ways in which the acknowledgement of those qualities can be used to refute global negative self-statements.

Challenging negative self-statements

Negative self-statements	Challenges
I'm no good at anything	I know I am a good gardener – I know I have patience and determination
I am not a good person	I look after my child – he seems to be getting on all right, so I must have instilled some good qualities

3. Feelings of powerlessness and vulnerability come from being unable to predict when an adverse reaction or depressed mood is likely to strike. Once other similar previously distressing situations are uncovered, it becomes easier to identify specific triggers that elicit high levels of distress. The identification of these cues can ameliorate feelings of helplessness in those stressful situations, especially if strategies to contain the occurrence of an adverse reaction can be employed at the outset.

4. Anxiety management strategies, such as slow breathing and imaginal techniques (e.g. imagining a walk on a beach or in a forest) can be used to control and reduce high levels of arousal which disrupt the use of other constructive coping strategies. For example, slow breathing while negotiating an upsetting situation can facilitate the concentration required to employ cognitive challenges.

Barriers to effective intervention

The uncensored disclosure of previous stressful events will only occur within a safe and supportive therapeutic environment and when rapport with the therapist has been established. Even then, the disclosure of traumatic past events may require several sessions to be fully discussed in terms of their influence on current stressors. It is also important to establish a mechanism by which new information and constructive experiences can be brought into the therapy situation to help change the way previously unpleasant events are interpreted.

The role of medication

Medication may be an adjunct to recovery in a percentage of individuals who have not responded, or only partially responded to intervention strategies as previously covered. Selective serotonin reuptake inhibitor (SSRI) antidepressants appear the most useful, by muting the intensity of depression and anxiety experienced by individuals. On rare occasions, medication may also assist pursuit of earlier 'lock' scenarios. For instance, one patient who, when depressed, ruminated about a pregnancy termination, 'remembered' certain sexual activities she had initiated as a child with her grandfather (and which had led to her pregnancy) only after commencing on an SSRI. The SSRI's effect was to mute her distress so that she could face remembering the events and was able to 'work through' their impact. Anxiolytic medications (e.g. benzodiazepines) are not recommended as a primary treatment however.

15

Chronic stress-related non-melancholic depression

Exposure to one or more uncontrollable stressors over an extended period of time can be associated with the development of non-melancholic depression. These stressors include chronic psychosocial adversity, physical illness, or exposure to recurrent psychological abuse and trauma. Unremitting and adverse life events can test the mettle of the most resilient individuals and exhaust their ability to adapt and cope.

At times, chronic stress-related depression may occur within the context of a history of early developmental deprivation. People who have had the misfortune to be exposed to early adversity may develop an expectation of further hardship and a pessimistic world view. Due to their long-standing experiences with uncontrollable and overwhelming stressors, such individuals may not have learnt effective problem-solving strategies to control or minimise the effects of future stressors.

The psychotransmitter model

Chronic and multiple salient and non-salient life events stimulate the production of large amounts of psychotransmitter which bombards the post-synaptic neuron and binds to receptor sites. Ion channels (perceptual and attributional biases) are stimulated to remain open, thus allowing the unremitting passage of ions into the neuron which, in turn, sets off numerous metabolic processes within the cell. Consequently, the neuron reacts to an unrelenting source of chronic stimulation and is flooded by the effects of high concentrations of intracellular chemical mediators (coping repertoires). These produce second messengers which carry with them the legacy of ineffective coping styles and a sense of mastery lost which, in turn, further anchors self-esteem in the off position making it less likely to overcome a depressive reaction even when negative life stressors cease and the individual experiences positive life events (Figs 15.1–15.4).

Fig. 15.1
Psychotransmitter
bombardment.

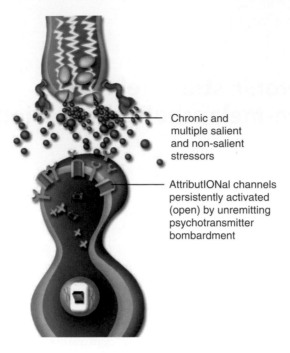

Chronic and
multiple salient
and non-salient
stressors

AttributIONal channels
persistently activated
(open) by unremitting
psychotransmitter
bombardment

Fig. 15.2 Chronic
activation of coping
repertoires.

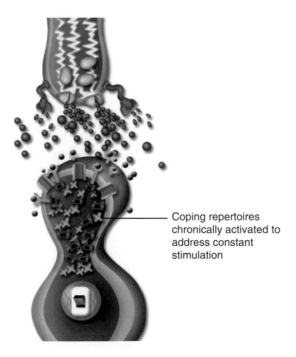

Coping repertoires
chronically activated to
address constant
stimulation

Fig. 15.3 Overarousal
and ineffectiveness
of coping repertoires.

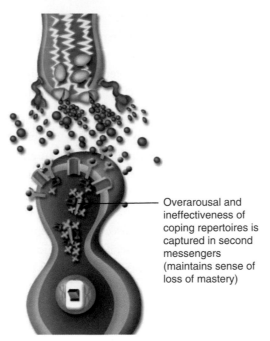

Overarousal and
ineffectiveness of
coping repertoires is
captured in second
messengers
(maintains sense of
loss of mastery)

Fig. 15.4 Self-esteem
anchored in the
off position.

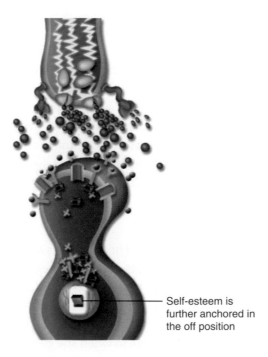

Self-esteem is
further anchored in
the off position

This model relies on the interplay of:
- Chronic psychotransmitter bombardment.
- Ion channels which remain open.
- Chronically activated protean defenses (e.g. coping repertoires).
- Processes that anchor self-esteem in the 'off' position.

Treatment strategies may involve using antagonists (such as pleasant events) to displace agonists (chronic stressors) from receptor sites and address the issues of open ion channels (change perceptual and attributional biases). Also, it may be necessary to re-train (using pleasurable activities) the neuron to respond to positive stimulation and thus reset the level of self-esteem. Other strategies, to be used in conjunction with the interventions described, may include 'turning off' the source of distressing psychotransmitters by removing the stressor. For example, if the chronic stressor happens to be an abusive husband, then the possibility of separation may need to be canvassed.

Case vignette – Julie

Julie, a 20-year-old single mother with two preschool-aged children, had been separated from her husband for 2 years. She and her children lived in a housing commission unit in an economically deprived region in the city. She had not completed high school nor obtained any further training and was only able to secure occasional casual work as a cashier at the local supermarket. Thus, she was constantly short of money, and trapped and exhausted by the responsibilities of looking after her children. Whenever her unemployed and frequently drunk husband dropped in to visit her and the children, there would be a verbal and/or physical altercation, leaving Julie feeling upset, angry, helpless and hopeless. He would sometimes inflict serious injuries which meant she would avoid seeing her mother and her friends, knowing they would comment on her bruises. Over the course of several months, Julie became progressively depressed and entertained thoughts of ending her life.

Case summary

Julie's feelings of helplessness and hopelessness about improving her living situation have prevented attempts at problem-solving. She is locked into a cycle of hardship, poverty and abuse, and her self-esteem and confidence have plummeted. In addition, her feelings of humiliation and shame have resulted in avoiding key sources of support (i.e. her mother and her friends). Thus Julie has few avenues to turn to when she gets overwhelmed and feels trapped – the only outlet she sees from her suffering is suicide.

Summary of Julie's problem areas

- Feelings of helplessness and hopelessness.
- Unfamiliarity with active problem-solving.
- Low self-esteem and self-confidence.
- Feelings of humiliation and shame.
- Feeling trapped by her many stressors.
- Suicidal ideation.

Principles of psychological intervention

The aim of therapy here is to help patients change their environment to minimise or eliminate stressors, or to empower them to overcome their stressors. In the short term, regular sessions of supportive counselling and active problem-solving strategies may be of assistance. In medium- to long-term therapy, individuals may benefit from learning how to actively challenge their negative self-perceptions and feelings of helplessness and hopelessness. Direct advice and instruction from the therapist can also be extremely helpful in facilitating the process of change.

A structure for psychological intervention
- Aim to reduce or eliminate exposure to psychosocial stressors.
- Supportive counselling and problem-solving strategies in the short term.
- Challenging negative self-perceptions in medium- to long-term therapy.
- Direct advice and instruction from the therapist.
- Suicide prevention strategies (e.g. contract-setting, crisis contact telephone numbers).

What sort of therapist?

A confident therapist who can work with the patient to engineer significant lifestyle changes and with a focus on practical problem-solving approaches is needed for this type of non-melancholic depressive disorder arising from chronic stressors. Building good rapport and a trusting, non-critical therapeutic relationship with the patient will also facilitate the process of making much-needed life changes.

Getting started

Establishing a mutual understanding of the level of chronic stress as well as the ways in which stressors interact with each other is an important starting point for psychological intervention. It may be necessary, if a point of crisis has been reached, to facilitate the physical removal of the patient from his or her environment in order to break the pattern of chronic stress, before starting a program of psychological intervention.

Establishing the areas for intervention

One way to determine the strategic areas for intervention is to examine long-term wishes and goals and telescope the patient's broad desires into short-term achievable plans. The technique described in the previous chapter on 'setting realistic goals' may be used in this context. Next, there needs to be mutual agreement about the main problem areas for intervention.

Problem area	Psychological intervention
• Feelings of helplessness and hopelessness	• Setting specific and achievable behavioural tasks
• Little or no active problem-solving	• Considering 'neutralising events' within a structured problem-solving and goal-setting framework
• Low self-esteem and self-confidence	• Cognitive therapy to raise self-esteem and self-confidence, and to learn to acknowledge successes
• Feeling trapped by lack of choices in dealing with stressors	• Supportive counselling and problem-solving to examine alternate choices

Intervention strategies

1. If the long-term goals are established at the outset of therapy, a logic for the course of therapy is imposed, and often very much appreciated by the patient. Within this framework, goals can be narrowed down to specific relevant and achievable behavioural tasks which challenge feelings of helplessness and hopelessness. Learning to 'engineer' regular positive experiences and making the environment more controllable and predictable can also lessen such feelings.

2. Before embarking on problem-solving strategies, it may first be necessary to clarify the problem. Often, chronic problems are deeply entwined with one another. Determining which of several problems need to be solved

first and determining the boundaries of each problem can require training in itself. Strategies for neutralising or removing the stressful life event can be worked into problem-solving strategies. For example, if the patient is desperately unhappy about staying with her husband and is on the cusp of leaving, the role of the therapist may be to promote and facilitate this process. Although the patient may experience difficulties at first, eventually they are available for a new and more satisfying relationship, and can be very appreciative of the support previously given by the therapist. In another example, a woman who was being subtly 'exploited' by her loving husband became severely depressed. Advising the husband to change his behaviour (and giving him good reasons for so doing) resulted in him apologising to his wife with the consequence that her depression lifted.

3. Cognitive challenges may be used to address issues of low self-esteem and self-confidence. One of the most common negative thinking styles that accompanies chronic stress-related depression is that of 'over-generalisation'.

Challenging negative thinking styles

Over-generalisations
For example,
'*My husband said I was "dumb" for not being able to fix the stove. He must be right.*'
'*I misunderstood the bank teller. I'm just dumb, I'll never understand anything.*'

The therapist's role is to challenge these over-generalisations by questioning whether failure at one or two tasks implies significant personal shortcomings. Challenging these thoughts also serves to negate other long-standing negative self-perceptions and to introduce the possibility of modifying thoughts and behaviours to reduce anxiety and distress.

It may also be useful to introduce the concept of self-reward to acknowledge small successes that would otherwise pass unnoticed. Self-reward may take the form of self-praise or engagement in pleasurable activities.

4. Supportive counselling needs to be used within the context of applying problem-solving strategies, some of which may require extensive planning and encouragement before they are attempted. The therapist's role may need to be broadened to that of mentor and case co-ordinator especially when major life decisions need to be enacted.

Barriers to effective intervention

The most likely barrier to change arises from the cumulative effects of multiple or ongoing chronic stressors impinging on the process of recovery from a depressive episode. If some of the key stressors are not removed or modified, then there is the risk of re-traumatisation or heightened sensitivity to those stressors, despite the beneficial effects of intervention in other areas.

The role of medication

A significant percentage of people who are depressed because of such chronic stressors receive some benefit, albeit not a cure, from selective serotonin reuptake inhibitor (SSRI) medication. While their problems remain, they are less preoccupied by them, and the greater distance is beneficial to them and to their mood state. Thus, such medication can be tested as a therapeutic component, but should not be viewed as the only therapy and is rarely the definitive approach. Again while other antidepressants are unlikely to be superior to SSRIs as a class, side-effect profiles (especially any impact on sleep) may dictate choice or trial of another drug class.

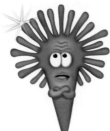

16

The perfectionist personality style and non-melancholic depression

Perfectionist personality style

There are many social advantages to possessing perfectionist personality characteristics. Hard working and ambitious, perfectionists are usually successful at any tasks they undertake. Their self-imposed high standards, self-discipline, and control usually ensure a high level of productivity and achievement. These personality features may lessen the likelihood of being exposed to and being overwhelmed by unexpected stressors. However, extreme manifestations of perfectionistic traits can result in indecisiveness or in behaviour patterns that are too rigid or controlling. For example, perfectionism may be displayed as a tendency to prevaricate on making the 'right' decision in a way that overshadows the more immediate demands of making a decision at all.

Key characteristics of the Perfectionist Personality Style (derived from our Temperament and Personality Questionnaire):
- Works hard at things.
- Tries to do everything well.
- Pushes themselves to be the best at things.
- Succeeds at most things.
- Commits fully to things.
- Works to full potential.

When stressors are either diverse, numerous, or excessive, features of the perfectionist personality style may be more of a hindrance than a help. Especially prone to self-criticism, individuals with features of this personality style, when overwhelmed by stress, may become locked into a destructive downward spiral of ruminations over past behaviours and future decision-making. Momentary respite from such distress is usually achieved by indulging in reckless behaviours (e.g. driving too fast or self-consolatory bingeing on comfort foods) which may, at best, only serve to defer addressing immediate stressors, and at worst, further exacerbate their impact.

It is uncommon for perfectionistic individuals to seek professional help unless coerced, for example, at the instigation of a frustrated partner or because of serious problems at work. When she or he does seek help, however, their critical style often poses a challenge for the therapist who has to meet the individual's exacting standards in order to win their confidence and build a sound therapeutic alliance.

Under stress the Perfectionist Personality Style is characterised by:
- Excessive ruminations over past behaviours and future decisions.
- Increased levels of self-criticism and a loss of pride.
- Behavioural paralysis due to indecision.
- Solace in comfort foods.

The psychotransmitter model

In our model, the saliency of stressors is driven by perceived threats to attain the 'ideal' outcome. Ion channels are selectively activated to filter information being processed by the neuron while problems in the efficient working of intracellular enzymes and proteins (early learning experiences, such as exposure to critical parenting, and other developmental factors) generate a 'harsh' neuronal system that works overtime to maintain self-regulation. Malfunctions at this level lead to the production of complex second messengers which incorporate feelings of ineffectiveness and which, in turn, switch off self-esteem, resulting in depression (Figs 16.1–16.4).

This model relies on the interplay of:
- Stressor saliency driven by threats to attain the 'ideal' outcome.
- Activation of selective attributIONal channels.
- Intracellular mediators which create a 'harsh' internal environment.
- Production of complex second messengers which switch off self-esteem.

To address this problem, one would have to examine attributional biases, early learning experiences and other developmental factors which shape cognitive schemas and coping repertoires. Practical strategies to promote and reward feelings of self-efficacy and self-mastery would also help to change the way in which potential stressors are perceived and handled.

Fig. 16.1 Stressor saliency driven by perceived threats and activation of selective attributIONal channels.

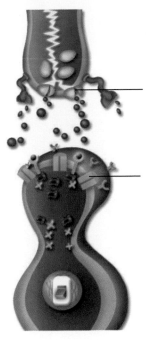

Saliency of stressor driven by perceived threats to attaining the 'ideal' ('falling short')

Activation of selective attributIONal channels filter information being processed

Fig. 16.2 Intracellular mediators create a 'harsh' internal environment.

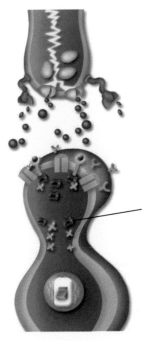

Intracellular mediators (e.g. exposure to critical parenting) create a 'harsh' internal environment ('try harder') and bind with salient aspects of the psychotransmitter

Fig. 16.3 Production of complex second messengers.

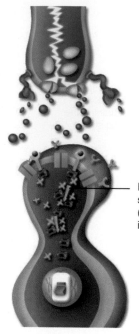

Production of complex second messengers (e.g. feelings of ineffectiveness)

Fig. 16.4 Second messengers switch off self-esteem.

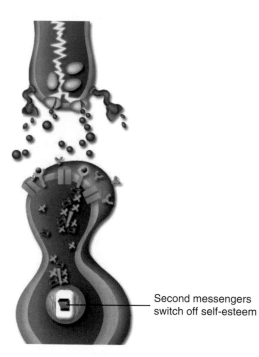

Second messengers switch off self-esteem

Case vignette – Susan

Susan is a 28-year-old single woman employed as a legal secretary in a large law firm in the city. Although she enjoyed her job, she felt anxious about the volume of work that she had to address to meet her own exacting standards. Susan began to doubt whether she could handle her workload and frequently dwelt on whether she was meeting her employer's expectations. She found herself staying back at work for several hours in order to complete her tasks to her satisfaction. With her spare time being eroded by the increasing demands at work, and her perception that her superior was suggesting that she was not performing to an appropriate standard, Susan found herself becoming stressed, depressed, and isolated. Her friendships suffered and her close friends became concerned for her well-being.

Over the course of several weeks, Susan's mood worsened. Her sleep was poor and she had little energy and motivation for activities that she usually enjoyed. Her level of concentration deteriorated at work, and Susan became increasingly self-critical and would often burst into tears. She tried to alleviate her sense of failure by spending more time alone at home after work, alternately bingeing on snack foods, or embarking on radical and stringent dietary restrictions to restore her sense of control over her life, at least for a while.

Case summary

Susan is spiralling into a depressive episode precipitated by her long-standing beliefs about her own abilities. Although her perfectionist personality style may have helped her achieve her goals, this same cognitive style and behaviour has obstructed her from overcoming her current stressors. She responds to stress by initially spending more time at work, sacrificing her recreational time, and the possibility of relief. Furthermore, because of her perfectionist personality style, it is highly unlikely that she would ever be satisfied with her level of work performance despite the extra hours that she puts in.

Dysfunctional thoughts, and attitudes towards others

- I have to be the best.
- Others are careless and unreliable.
- It's a disaster when things go wrong.
- I can only rely on myself to do things well.

Summary of Susan's problem areas

- Excessive rumination over perceived mistakes.
- High levels of self-criticism because of perceived incompetence.

- Low sense of self-efficacy.
- 'Black-and-white' thinking.
- Little acknowledgement of achievements.

Principles of psychological intervention

Medium- to long-term intervention of 12 to 20 sessions over a 6-month period, with a strong task-oriented focus, can be helpful for individuals with features of this personality style. The immediate aims of therapy would be to help them regain a sense of control and mastery over their environment. Psychological strategies such as active problem-solving techniques and goal-setting skills which promote a strong sense of self-efficacy at the outset are desirable, as they build on existing strengths and natural inclinations.

In long-term therapy it is necessary to address the core issues of this personality style that ultimately lead to problems: perceived imperfections in themselves or in others; intolerance of others' mistakes or transgressions; difficulties in completing tasks which are 'less than perfect'; and difficulties with relinquishing control to others when appropriate. A narrative approach may be useful to elicit and clarify how perfectionist attitudes and behaviours have shaped their life experiences and life course. Discussion of early experiences that may have also shaped such attitudes and behaviours, for example, growing up with highly critical or demanding parents, can help the development of insight into the origins of their personality style and help facilitate attitudinal and behavioural change.

Reckless or self-consolatory behaviours, unless dangerous or demeaning, should not be the primary focus of psychological intervention but rather serve as a barometer of distress during the course of therapy.

A structure for psychological intervention
- Medium- to long-term therapy.
- Focus on tasks and clearly defined outcomes.
- Intervention strategies such as structured problem-solving and goal-setting may be helpful in the short term.
- Long-term intervention strategies need to target the core features of self-criticism, intolerance, and procrastination.
- Reckless or self-consolatory behaviours should not be the primary focus of intervention.

What sort of therapist?

Open and clear communication by the therapist is crucial to the success of building a good therapeutic alliance. Individuals with perfectionist characteristics are likely to be just as critical towards their therapist as they are to themselves and others. So the ideal therapist will possess a combination of efficiency, purposefulness, and clarity in communication style, together with sound judgement in providing encouragement and support when required. Gains may also be achieved with a therapist who can model a 'light' (without being facile) approach to addressing problem areas, as people with predominant features of a perfectionistic style may be prone to taking themselves and life events far 'too seriously'.

Getting started

What are the aims of therapy? This has to be jointly established by therapist and patient at the start of any psychological intervention. A useful strategy is to set a framework for understanding the development of present difficulties from the patient's point of view. This can be achieved by charting a timeline of significant life events that relate to the development or manifestations of

---

Establishing a framework for therapy

Draw a vertical line with the periods 'childhood', 'adolescence and early adulthood', and 'adulthood' clearly marked. Next, indicate on the line events that are highly significant to the patient and/or relevant to the development of current difficulties while asking about the significance of those events.

├ Childhood
  Anxiety about going to school; bullied at school.
  Parents separated and divorced.
├ Adolescence
  Tried drugs; no friends.
├ Early adulthood
  Attended one year of university then dropped out; unemployed for several years.
  Break up of relationship of 3 years.
├ Adulthood
  Difficulties with current relationship; difficulties getting on with people at work.

features of this personality style. This could be combined with a narrative approach and the use of 'deconstructive questioning' (listed in Chapter 12). Describing how thoughts, attitudes and behaviours surrounding previous significant events relate to current difficulties helps to clarify the role and impact of perfectionist traits. Once documented, it may be easier to determine and negotiate the aims of therapy from both the patient's and the therapist's perspectives to arrive at a mutually agreeable therapeutic contract.

Establishing the areas for intervention

A technique which is helpful for setting specific targets for change is that of asking the patient what they would like to be different in their life. An example of this type of questioning is derived from motivational interviewing techniques (Ivey, 1988; Miller & Rollnick, 1991). The 'miracle question' takes the form of '… if you went to sleep tonight and, as you slept, a miracle occurred in your life so that all your immediate problems would be solved, how would your life be different the next day when you wake up? How would you know it was different?' Next, draw up a plan for intervention, such as the one below, which incorporates several important psychological intervention strategies.

Problem area	Psychological intervention
• Excessive ruminations over past behaviours and future decisions	• Thought stopping and distraction techniques
• Increased levels of self-criticism and self-blame	• Cognitive challenge of dysfunctional thoughts
• Behavioural paralysis by indecision	• Structured problem-solving and goal-setting skills
• Lowered sense of self-efficacy	• Setting specific and achievable behavioural tasks
• Poor self-reward skills	• Teaching how to self-reward
• Poor tolerance for perceived 'sub-optimal' performance	• Desensitisation to perceived 'imperfections'

Intervention strategies

1. Thought stopping and distraction techniques aim to halt the rapid succession of dysfunctional thoughts that lead to or exacerbate a depressive episode. Active thought stopping and distraction comprise two separate strategies which can be used consecutively. The first technique, thought stopping, involves using a 'cognitive block', for example, visualising a huge 'STOP' sign or whistling, to re-focus attention away from dysfunctional

thoughts. The second strategy, distraction, may involve a number of different mental tasks depending on individual preference. Examples of such tasks are:

- reciting the alphabet backwards;
- thinking of as many adjectives as possible beginning with the letter 'B';
- trying to spell backwards complex words like 'supercilious';
- visualising a pleasant and engaging scene such as a holiday destination.

2. Challenging dysfunctional cognitions can be used to address excessive and irrational self-criticism and self-blame.

Challenging dysfunctional cognitions

Saturday, 10 March

Situation: Missing a train home from the city.

Feelings: Angry, upset with self for not checking timetable.

Thoughts: 'I am so careless', 'I'm always so disorganised'.

Challenges: 'I am usually aware of the train timetable. Missing one train does not make me careless or disorganised.'

Alternate interpretation: 'I must have had something on my mind to forget the train time. It doesn't really matter if I am a bit late getting home anyway.'

3. Structured problem-solving and goal-setting skills are two strategies which together can restore a sense of control and mastery, and address the anxiety over decision-making that is characteristic. Structured problem-solving involves:

- deciding on a specific problem to address,
- brainstorming possible solutions,
- rating or ranking the possible solutions,
- deciding on the 'best' solution or combination of solutions,
- implementing the solution (within a specified time frame),
- reviewing the success of the solution.

Perfectionist individuals often judge that there are only two options for resolving a current crisis. They often create a 'stable unstable' situation, 'unstable' because when they are moving towards one option, the other option looks more attractive and they move back, with the 'stable' oscillations ensuring no forward progress. A key strategy is to brainstorm 3-to-6 solutions rather than the black-and-white option of two. Some perfectionistic depressed people see only one option: which may be to kill themselves; here, the need to identify and consider multiple options is even more immediate.

Goal-setting helps focus attention on future plans and how those plans may be achieved. Setting long-term (5–10 years) and short-term (3–12 months) goals helps discourage excessive preoccupation with decision-making. Goals may be further subdivided into separate domains such as 'social', 'occupational', or 'personal' goals to ensure representation across several facets of lifestyle.

4. The exercise of setting specific and achievable behavioural tasks may be used to enhance self-esteem and self-efficacy and provide clear indices for success in overcoming problems. The strategy aims to capitalise on other attributes that may be overlooked or ignored.

Example of setting specific and achievable behavioural tasks

- Make a list of key personality attributes.
- Focus on two or three of these personality attributes.
- Develop a behavioural plan around these personality attributes.

For example:

- A good sense of humour could be operationalised into organising a regular group of friends to go out to comedy shows or humourous movies.
- Sociability could be operationalised into initiating regular social outings with friends, or initiating a pleasant conversation with a stranger.
- Artistic ability could be developed by attending regular art classes.

---

5. Encourage the use of self-reward to help acknowledge positive behavioural changes which would otherwise pass unnoticed. For example, being able to distract from dysfunctional self-critical thoughts could be rewarded by a small treat. Graphical representation of success such as a 'star chart' or other device can also serve to help implement and sustain change.

6. Desensitisation to perceived imperfections, both in themselves and in others. Exposure and desensitisation to mild levels of perceived 'disorganisation' or loss of control can help build resilience to such stressors. This may involve creating a hierarchy of 'disorganisation', rating events or tasks from the easiest to the most difficult to tolerate. Next, implement a structured program of graduated exposure, while maintaining a low level of anxiety and arousal. Examples of such tasks could include taking a different route home from work twice a week, 'wasting' time watching

television instead of engaging in more productive tasks, or writing a letter to a close friend with the non-dominant hand.

Building resilience

To develop resilience to further depressive episodes, it is necessary to define and strengthen an individual's sense of 'self' which is independent of their achievements or of other's perceptions of them. One strategy is to list and discuss positive and negative attributes which are not related to perfectionism, such as a good sense of humour, or a caring nature, together with specific examples of situations in which those attributes manifest.

It can also be extremely useful to have the individual view themselves as others see them, in order to understand the impact their behaviours have on the people around them. Role plays or videotapes help self-reflection on perfectionist traits that impact on their interactions with others.

Lastly, behavioural experiments can be set up which challenge dysfunctional cognitive schemas about the world and their place in it. For example, a cognitive schema that 'people are only going to remember my faults' could be challenged by asking others whether they remember specific incidents in which the individual's perceived flaws were highlighted.

Barriers to effective intervention

Despite the best plans and therapeutic strategies, there may still be barriers to achieving success. For example, there may be lack of recognition of the key problem areas (i.e. perfectionism) by the patient. Instead the patient's focus may be directed elsewhere. Thus, a therapist will have to thoroughly discuss the aims of therapy before embarking on an intervention program for an individual with perfectionist personality traits.

The role of medication

Both formal studies (e.g. Zuroff et al., 2000) and clinical experience suggest that individuals with a perfectionistic personality and non-melancholic depression are less likely to respond to antidepressant medication. Firstly, such individuals like to be in control and do not readily surrender control to others, or to medication. Secondly, their depression is generally more underpinned by a sense of failing to meet standards or goals (a very cognitive feature) rather than emotional dysregulation. Thirdly, there is difficulty in their trusting that medication will assist, and that the therapist is going to be truly useful, so that difficulties in forming a treatment alliance reduces the chance of responding. Fourthly, the need for 'control' acts against any propensity for spontaneous remission and improvement, thus weakening a possible springboard for a more definitive response to therapy.

If antidepressant medication is to be trialled, it is best to suggest to the patient that it is viewed as an adjunct and not the main approach, to pre-empt the disappointment (showed by the patient and the therapist) when medication fails.

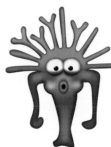

17

The irritable personality style and non-melancholic depression

Irritable personality style

People with features of an irritable personality style are usually quick-tempered and volatile. They may be like this all the time, or pleasant when life is calm and only irritable when stressed. They make their displeasure known to all around by flaring up but settling down once they have expressed themselves. Life with someone with irritable traits can be an emotional roller-coaster of brief and intense periods of anger followed by more peaceful episodes of calm. People with irritable traits usually suffer from high levels of ambient autonomic arousal and can be quite grumpy, especially when under stress. In their day-to-day dealings with others, such as colleagues at work, friends and family members, they may be highly respected and well liked. They may also tend to feel remorseful, and regret the 'collateral' damage they cause to the psychological well-being of those around them.

Characteristics of the Irritable Personality Style (derived from our Temperament and Personality Questionnaire):
- Hot-tempered and loses control when stressed.
- Snaps at others when irritated.
- Gets cranky with themselves and with others.
- Impatient.
- Stresses easily.
- Easily rattled.

High levels of autonomic arousal together with low frustration tolerance drives the explosive fractiousness and anger which characterise this personality style. Secondary problems arising from such behaviours such as social isolation, loneliness, and interpersonal problems with colleagues at work or family members are common.

Often, individuals with an irritable personality style will seek help at the instigation of family members who bear the brunt and suffer the consequences of their angry outbursts. Although professional help is unlikely to be sought directly for the underlying temperamental and personality characteristics of heightened arousal and low frustration tolerance, these issues nevertheless need to be heeded when developing an effective program of psychological intervention. The focus of therapy, however, needs to be on alleviating the distress associated with the 'collateral' problems that often precipitate and maintain depressive episodes.

Under stress the Irritable Personality Style is characterised by:
- Brief uncontrollable outbursts of anger.
- Being snappy at people.
- Lashing out at others.
- Being impatient with him/herself.

The psychotransmitter model

Our model here is of a neuron that for most of the time functions well (self-esteem is switched on) despite an innate propensity for excitability (high levels of ambient arousal). However, when over stimulated, cellular processes go awry partly because cellular functioning is already 'close to the edge' (the individual is often 'edgy'). The threat to self-esteem causes feedback which, adversely, increases the level of neuronal stimulation. In our neurotransmitter analogy, specific types of psychotransmitters (specific types of life events or stressors) act on the greater innate excitability of the neuron. Intracellular mediators (defences and coping repertoires) become overwhelmed by the increasing level of neuronal activity resulting in a spiral of ever-increasing excitation until the energy is discharged in epochs of 'crabbiness', 'irritability', or 'anger'. Cognitive appraisal of these irritable outbursts modify the quality of second messengers (e.g. awareness of being viewed as unpleasant) which switch off self-esteem and causes depression (Figs 17.1–17.4).

This model relies on the interplay of:
- A propensity within the neuron towards excitation.
- Overactivity of intracellular processes.
- Increasing levels of neuronal excitation which result in energy surges.
- Feedback about energy surges which modifies quality of second messengers.
- Self-esteem being switched off.

Treatment strategies would need to address the way in which neuronal excitability spirals out of control. Strategies that help to decrease neuronal excitability, by reducing overall arousal (e.g. meditation, relaxation therapy)

Fig. 17.1 A propensity within the neuron towards excitation.

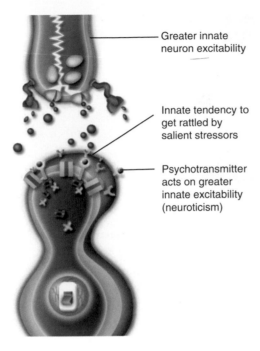

Greater innate neuron excitability

Innate tendency to get rattled by salient stressors

Psychotransmitter acts on greater innate excitability (neuroticism)

Fig. 17.2 Overactivity of intracellular processes.

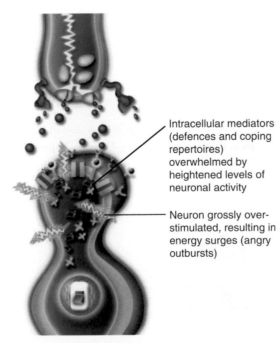

Intracellular mediators (defences and coping repertoires) overwhelmed by heightened levels of neuronal activity

Neuron grossly over-stimulated, resulting in energy surges (angry outbursts)

Fig. 17.3 Cognitive
appraisal of irritable
outbursts modify the
quality of second
messengers.

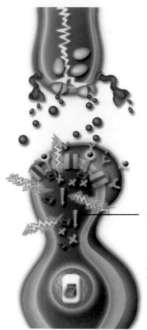

Cognitive appraisal of
irritable outbursts modify
the quality of second
messengers (e.g.
awareness of being
viewed as unpleasant)

Fig. 17.4 Switching
off of self-esteem.

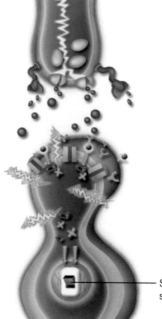

Second messengers
switch off self-esteem

or by modulating excitation by encouraging the recognition of negative feedback (anger management) are helpful. In addition, other strategies which help to attenuate receptor sensitivity to certain types of psychotransmitters (stressors such as being kept waiting) may help to control over-stimulation.

Case vignette – Andrew

Andrew had single-handedly built up a highly successful construction company which now had offices in five capital cities. He is married with two adult children who recently moved away from home and, at the age of 56 years, was looking forward to a comfortable retirement at 60 years. Despite his professional and personal achievements, Andrew had always suffered from symptoms of anxiety and described himself as a somewhat nervy person. He had a good professional and personal relationship with most of his staff, but was prone to bouts of extreme anger when frustrated by events at work or when he was busy and overworked. Often he would expect his staff to understand his needs and 'read his mind', getting irritated when they could not fulfil his expectations. When he was very upset, his outbursts usually took the form of yelling at staff, or criticising them for not performing well enough.

When stressed, he would also lash out at home at his wife, who bore the brunt of his anger and irritability. He would also spend lavishly and impulsively on novel electronic gadgets for his home and office, and frequently lost considerable sums betting on horse races. When particularly stressed, Andrew would spend several hours at the bar opposite his office and not go home till very late. His friends and family were often upset with his angry outbursts and he found himself becoming increasingly socially isolated. His wife had threatened to leave him on several occasions. Andrew had begun to feel that others did not understand him and, as time wore on, became increasingly depressed as he struggled to maintain his work commitments and save his marriage.

Case summary

Andrew's depressive episode has been precipitated by the damage inflicted on his work and personal life by his emotional volatility. These secondary issues include the financial stressors imposed by his impulsive spending, a lack of social support, and the strains of his marriage, all of which have significantly contributed to his immediate distress and exacerbated his anxiety, irritability, and reactivity to further stress. Furthermore, his expectation that others should be able to understand his needs and 'read his mind' has accelerated his downward spiral and he is at risk of a serious episode of clinical depression.

Dysfunctional thoughts and attitudes

- Others really irritate me.
- I am unable to control my temper.
- I cannot control my level of stress.

Summary of Andrew's problem areas

- Heightened levels of anxiety and stress.
- Low frustration tolerance.
- Poor communication skills.
- Problems in social, professional, and personal relationships.
- Dysfunctional behaviours when stressed.

Principles of psychological intervention

Structured short-term interventions of up to eight sessions which focus on specific problem areas and clear benchmarks for improvement will be helpful, together with anxiety-reduction strategies. Group-based interventions have a role if they encourage disclosure of stressful events and cause reflection on the impact of explosive anger on lifestyle and on other people.

As they have a low tolerance to frustration, it may be useful to initially focus on strategies which produce immediate relief and small but rapid improvements, for example, encouraging the individual to embark on a program of vigorous exercise. Individuals with features of this personality style are likely to comply with structured homework assignments, reading material, and other tasks, provided that these bring about noticeable improvements in mood and stress levels, and they are also likely to be compliant with antidepressant medication.

If there are serious secondary problems with other people such as their spouse, family members or close friends, it may be prudent to include them in the process of therapy, especially where such involvement can significantly influence the recovery process.

A structure for psychological intervention
- Short-term intervention.
- Focus on specific problem areas with clear goals for therapy.
- Initial focus of therapy on anxiety reduction and later on strategies for curbing irritability.

- Strategies which provide immediate or rapid relief at the start of therapy.
- Use homework tasks and reading material to consolidate gains made during therapy sessions.

What sort of therapist?

The ideal therapist is one who is able to communicate in a clear and straightforward manner and who is able to help address immediate problems, while being mindful of underlying personality features which have contributed to the development of the depressive episode. Individuals with an irritable personality style are also likely to become irritable and angry with their therapist during the course of therapy, necessitating the need for a 'strong' therapist who will not be intimidated by the ventilation of strong emotion. Episodes of anger or irritability during the sessions may be used to model more appropriate expressions of frustration or dissatisfaction.

Getting started

Establishing a framework for therapy may include setting firm limits for expressions of anger. An analysis of how irritable personality features have contributed to the client's present problems, and negotiation of those aspects of their present difficulties to be addressed in therapy, is also needed.

Establishing a framework for therapy
A two-stage process
1. 'Damage control' incorporating techniques that will help remedy or contain problems that are a consequence of irritability and explosive anger.
2. Prevention of further disruptions to lifestyle, by learning strategies to minimise the likelihood of angry outbursts.

Establishing the areas for intervention

By the time such patients present for treatment, high levels of arousal together with ongoing serious lifestyle problems will have exacerbated an already volatile temperament. An initial strategy would be to reduce arousal before prioritising problem areas. If possible, enlist the support of spouses, partners, or parents who can share responsibility and help diffuse potentially stressful situations.

Next, document specific problems and consider psychological interventions that address these issues:

Problem area	Psychological intervention
• Heightened levels of arousal and increased sensitivity to stressful events	• Relaxation training and slow-breathing skills, vigorous exercise
• Social, personal, and professional relationship problems due to irritability and anger expression	• Relationship counselling, strategies to mend rifts in social, personal, and professional relationships
• Low frustration tolerance	• Graded exposure to frustration and desensitisation
• Difficulties with the appropriate expression of displeasure or distress	• Role play, modelling
• Limited and dysfunctional behavioural repertoires, such as lashing out at others when stressed	• Anger management, conflict resolution skills, assertiveness training

Intervention strategies

1. Relaxation training and slow-breathing techniques are used to help reduce high levels of arousal, and hypersensitivity to stress. Progressive muscle relaxation, practised twice a day, may reduce day-to-day autonomic arousal. This may be coupled with slow-breathing strategies, to be used to quickly reduce arousal when a blow-up is likely to occur. The concentration and time required to practise these exercises may be too great for some, and thus compliance in using them too low to be effective. An alternative strategy is an exercise program of brisk walking, jogging, or running.
   • Progressive muscle relaxation.
   • Slow-breathing exercises.
   • Vigorous exercise.
2. Relationship counselling and strategies to address problems in social relationships need to be implemented early (if applicable) as these stressors can impact on the effectiveness of other psychological strategies. It may be

necessary to conduct joint sessions with a spouse or partner to discuss the aims and progress of therapy as well as to facilitate more effective communication. A discussion of ways in which problems and previous rifts in relationships with work colleagues, friends, and other family members can be constructively addressed, may be needed.

3. Graded exposure to planned frustrations can be a useful way to 'desensitise' to such situations and to practise anxiety-reduction skills. Develop a list of potentially frustrating situations which may be controlled and modified to some extent. Follow with exposure to these situations, and then document initial reactions, and the outcome of implementing specific anxiety-reduction techniques.

List of potentially frustrating situations
- Taking a different route while driving home from work in peak hour.
- Waiting in a queue at the bank or at the supermarket at lunchtime.
- Being put on 'hold' while trying to speak to someone on the telephone.
- Not commenting when provoked by a workmate's regular critical comments about others.
- Supporting and watching a losing sporting team.

4. Role plays and modelling of more appropriate expression of displeasure or distress can help skills to generalise to situations outside therapy sessions. Using a previously unpleasant incident at work or at home can provide the necessary material to role play and to model with the therapist more appropriate expressions of anger and frustration.

Key elements of the role play or modelling experience
It includes:
- A clear and concise account of the original incident, including outcomes.
- Detailed analysis of the concomitant physical and emotional experiences as the incident unfolded.
- An account of how the situation could have been better dealt with using more appropriate expression of anger or frustration.
- Modelling or role playing the desired outcome with the therapist.

5. Anger management techniques, conflict resolution skills, and assertiveness training are strategies which can replace previous dysfunctional
expressions of anger and frustration. Anger management encompasses a
number of related techniques which help identify specific events that
trigger angry reactions, common ways of reacting to anger and frustration, and methods by which such responses can be curbed or modified.
Conflict resolution offers skills dealing with interpersonal conflicts and
difficulties. Assertiveness training directly addresses skills' deficits in the
expression of negative emotions.

Skills training

a) *Anger management techniques* identify specific triggers, common or
habitual ways of expressing anger and frustration, and methods to
change destructive behaviours.
b) *Conflict resolution skills* teach how to deal with interpersonal
conflicts and difficulties, using a number of cognitive and
behavioural strategies.
c) *Assertiveness training* addresses skills' deficits in the expression of
anger and frustration.

Building resilience

For this personality style, building resilience can be assisted by deconstructing stressors into their component parts so they are not so overwhelming. Learning to analyse components of life stressors and how they
impact on self-esteem can assist in lessening impact. Learning to 'isolate' or
'quarantine' stressors can help the individual to preserve their self-esteem
and sense of self-efficacy as well as learning to tolerate frustration without
'blowing up'.

Barriers to effective intervention

Though these strategies may be highly effective, they are only useful if practised over a long period of time. Compliance with treatment can be difficult
with individuals who have irritable personality features because of their
impatience and poor frustration tolerance, which also makes them vulnerable to set-backs during therapy. The role of the therapist is not only to

provide the necessary psychological skills but to help maintain motivation in the face of set-backs during the course of therapy.

The role of medication

If irritability is, as commonly thought, a reflection of high-externalised trait anxiety, then the underlying 'emotional dysregulation' contributing to the depression will generally respond significantly to a selective serotonin reuptake inhibitor (SSRI) antidepressant and to some other antidepressant classes that have anxiety-reduction properties. If the irritability is not driven by anxiety, the antidepressant medication will be less likely to be effective.

For some individuals, SSRI medication will be sufficient in and of itself but, for many people, non-medication techniques detailed above are preferred – alone, or in conjunction with SSRI medication.

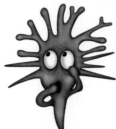

18

The anxious worrying personality style and non-melancholic depression

Anxious worrying personality style

While many people experience periods of worry in their lives, those with an anxious worrying temperament have a tendency to worry most of the time, seemingly over the most trivial incidents and situations. They are often described by others as being 'highly strung' or 'nervy'. Domains of anxiety may include worrying that the worst will happen even after minor events, being especially sensitive about unexpected changes in their immediate environment, and getting upset over minor things that go wrong. People with this type of temperament are easily upset and stressed, and can seem tense and jumpy. When distressed, they tend to find comfort in talking to close friends about their worries and in seeking reassurance, or going quiet and keeping to themselves. Sometimes they may resort to temporary relief from their worries by engaging in pleasurable activities as a means of distraction.

Key characteristics of the Anxious Worrying Temperament (derived from our Temperament and Personality Questionnaire):
- High levels of autonomic arousal.
- Easily rattled and upset.
- Tense and nervy.
- Worry over minor things.
- Take things too personally.
- Worry that the worst will happen.

When stressed, key personality features of the anxious worrier, such as ruminative and catastrophic thoughts, worsen. When such thoughts begin to focus on excessive self-doubt, and pessimism about the future, together with a sense of ineffectiveness or helplessness, a depressive episode may arise. Depression and anxiety may assume a cyclical pattern with one following and exacerbating the symptoms of the other. In the short term, people with features of this personality style may seek advice and reassurance from others. Although they may derive some immediate comfort and relief from their distress by discussing their worries with family members and friends, they may repeatedly need to address the same concerns as worries keep re-surfacing. In the long term, their confidants may tire of such high levels of tension and reassurance seeking. If family and friends withdraw support or are unavailable, this can further exacerbate depression and worry.

People with features of this personality style are likely to seek help from mental health professionals, especially when their excessive worry becomes overwhelming and/or their usual supports are unavailable. They are likely to be highly motivated to seek relief from their chronic worry which many recognise as a risk factor to their depressive episodes. However, there is a danger that help-seeking may become an extension of their repertoire of reassurance-seeking behaviours, especially when family and friends are unavailable.

Under stress the Anxious Worrying Personality Style is characterised by:
- Ruminative and catastrophic thoughts.
- Self-doubt and pessimism about the future.
- Sense of ineffectiveness or helplessness.
- Heightened levels of anxiety.
- Reassurance-seeking from others.

The psychotransmitter model

This personality style is characterised by high levels of arousal or neuroticism (the neuron is primed for affective dysregulation), and chronic levels of worry, indicated by negative perceptual and attributional styles (faulty ion channels). Our model favours notions of high receptor sensitivity, as well as ion channels which are frequently open to allow the free exchange of ions between the cell membrane and the extracellular space. Stimulation by the neurotransmitter docking on the receptor results in a series of chemical reactions which reverberate throughout the neuron and are amplified by the neuron's propensity to be dysregulated. Faulty ion channels (faulty perceptions and attributional styles) and the overactivation of intracellular enzymes (negative cognitive schemas) also serve to keep the level of overall excitability high. Second messengers, which incorporate aspects of the stressor and entrenched cognitive schemas, switch off self-esteem resulting in depression (Figs 18.1–18.4).

In this instance, raising the level of excitability (arousal) to increase self-esteem will possibly be detrimental to the neuron, while immediately lowering the level of excitability will lessen the likelihood of self-esteem being compromised.

Fig. 18.1 Greater
neuronal excitability
and an overinclusive
saliency mechanism.

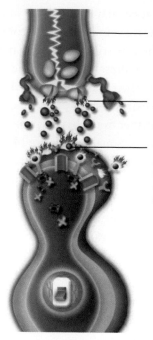

Greater innate
neuron excitability

Overinclusive
saliency mechanism
magnifies the impact
of stressors

Psychotransmitter
acts on greater
innate excitability
(neuroticism) of the
neuron

Fig. 18.2 Faulty ion
channels and over-
activation of negative
cognitive schemas.

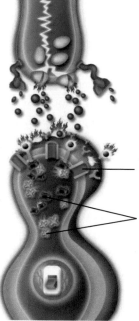

AttributIONal
channels wide open

Overactivation of
negative cognitive
schemas (doubts
about mastery and
control)

Fig. 18.3 Production
of complex second
messengers.

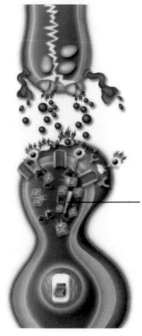

Production of complex
second messenger
incorporating aspects of
the stressor and
entrenched cognitive
schemas

Fig. 18.4 Processes
that switch off
self-esteem.

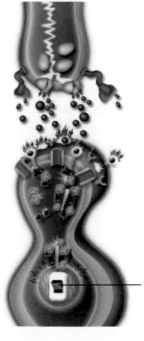

Self-esteem is
switched off by
second messengers

This model relies on the interplay of:
• A propensity within the neuron for excitation.
• Faulty ion channels.
• Overactivation of intracellular enzymes.
• Production of complex second messengers.
• Processes that interfere with self-esteem regulation.

Treatment strategies aim to change the excitation 'set-point' of the neuron so that lower levels of stimulation may restore self-esteem. However, the issue of faulty ion channels (faulty perceptual and attributional biases) and overactive intracellular enzymes (negative cognitive schemas) will simultaneously need to be addressed to break the cycle of heightened excitation.

Case vignette – Louise

As far back as Louise could remember she had always been a worrier. Her mother had often commented on how Louise, as a child, 'stressed out' over the slightest incidents such as whether she was going to be on time for school if the school bus was slightly late or whether her friends liked her as much as they said they did. Her worries continued now that she was in her 40s, divorced and mother to three school-age children. Louise worried about whether her children were studying hard enough, whether she was a good enough mother, and whether she could eventually return to part-time secretarial work. She would often worry about the worst possible events that could happen, and as a result, was often easily upset and appeared tense, nervy, and moody to her friends. She had a close friend to whom she would regularly speak on the telephone and discuss her problems and seek reassurance. Sometimes she would go out to dinner at the local club with her girlfriends to take her mind off her problems. When her usual outlets for stress-relief were unavailable, Louise became increasingly anxious and distressed. More recently, she had begun to get depressed as her numerous worries, despite reassurances from her friends, threatened to overwhelm her.

Case summary

Louise has a long history of chronic worry, to some extent modified by her habit of seeking reassurance via her friends. She constantly entertains 'catastrophic' worries that the worst will happen. Relying on her friends' reassurances and on distraction as a method of overcoming her anxieties has prevented her from developing any effective personal method to manage and reduce her level of stress. Over time, she has been overwhelmed by multiple stressors, and her usual coping mechanisms have become ineffective.

Dysfunctional thoughts and attitudes

- The world is a dangerous place.
- No matter how hard I plan, things always go wrong.
- It is a disaster when events do not go to plan.
- I need someone to reassure me that everything is all right.

Summary of Louise's problem areas

- Overgeneralisation and catastrophic thoughts.
- Coping behaviours that do not directly address her worries.
- Lifestyle shaped around her anxieties.
- Succumbing to worries when usual outlets for stress release are unavailable.

Principles of psychological intervention

Various types of psychological and alternate interventions, especially those that serve to decrease arousal levels and reduce stress, may be effective with people who have features of an anxious worrying personality style. Basic stress management skills, hypnotherapy, relaxation, meditation, and regular exercise will all help to reduce arousal levels and hence decrease symptom severity. Other forms of cognitive therapy would be helpful in order to address the dysfunctional and long-standing thinking styles that accompany this type of personality profile. It is likely that people with characteristics of anxious worrying will be easier to engage in therapy compared to those with other personality features, as they may be more motivated to find 'solutions' to their worries (and as they are keen to seek help and support from a therapist).

It is possible to treat such individuals in small groups with a structured therapy format. A group format not only provides a supportive milieu in which to disclose and challenge irrational or unrealistic catastrophic worries, but others in the group can provide a social support network. Booster sessions may need to be offered in the long term to consolidate gains made in initial treatment.

A structure for psychological intervention
- Highly structured psychological intervention.
- Individual or group intervention.
- Focus on specific strategies for reducing autonomic arousal.
- Address dysfunctional thinking styles.
- Booster sessions to consolidate gains.

What sort of therapist?

Depressed clients with an anxious worrying personality style benefit from a therapist who can impose a structure on the psychological intervention without getting sidetracked by the client's need for reassurance and support. Although the therapist may demonstrate interest in the nature of a client's worries, the therapist may need to maintain a degree of emotional distance in order to help challenge their client's irrational cognitive schemas.

Getting started

By the time such clients present for treatment, they are likely to feel overwhelmed by and ineffective in their day-to-day activities. In developing a psychological intervention program, it would be important to validate some of their concerns while suggesting some simple strategies for minimising the level of stress. It could be useful to start with grouping some of the key domains of concern into broad categories, each of which can be managed at a practical level.

Grouping the major domains of concern

Family	Personal	Work related
Children's schoolwork	Need to go for a checkup	Inability to work overtime
Elderly parents	No time for holidays	Financial difficulties
Quality of relationship with husband		

It may be easier to address such concerns in groups with strategies aimed at targeting the major issues in each domain. For example, the main concern in the 'Family' domain may be related to lack of time to spend with the family. Suggesting some time-management strategies, such as scheduling regular family outings or daily 'family time', may alleviate some of the more immediate stresses that contribute towards feeling overwhelmed by such worries. Personal stressors are largely related to not finding time for oneself or attending to one's needs. Strategies that help to prioritise tasks and challenge notions of putting others' needs before one's own may be helpful here. Suggested options for either improving their financial position or living within the constraints of a tight budget would be helpful to address this particular constellation of worries.

Establishing the areas for intervention

It is especially important to systematically note potential problem areas for clients with this personality style prior to commencing treatment, as they may otherwise become overwhelmed by a multitude of worries. Organising and prioritising areas of concern at the outset of therapy assists with basic time management and goal-setting which are useful skills in stress management.

Problem area	Psychological intervention
• Heightened levels of autonomic arousal and limited skills in arousal modulation	• Relaxation training and slow breathing skills, light exercise
• Distorted thinking styles including catastrophic thinking, overgeneralisation and lack of reality-testing	• Cognitive challenges to distorted thinking styles, and behavioural experiments
• Low sense of self-efficacy, confidence, and mastery over life events	• Graded exposure to goal-oriented and pleasurable tasks, documenting achievements, and using self-reward
• Poor problem-solving skills	• Breaking problems into manageable components and structured problem-solving skills
• Poor goal-setting and time-management skills	• Goal-setting and time-management skills
• Reliance on others for reassurance	• Gradually learning to tolerate and overcome discomfort rather than seeking reassurance

Intervention strategies

1. Heightened levels of autonomic arousal may be addressed by strategies such as progressive muscle relaxation (described previously), meditation techniques, and slow breathing exercises. Physical exercises such as *Tai Chi* or yoga can also reduce high levels of arousal.

2. Cognitive challenges can be used to address dysfunctional or irrational thinking styles. In addition, a series of behavioural experiments are useful for challenging specific thinking styles, such as 'catastrophising' (e.g. 'everything is a disaster and I won't be able to cope'), 'overgeneralising' (e.g. 'I couldn't find my glasses today. I'm always losing things') or 'black and white thinking' (e.g. 'My son got into a fight today at school. This whole day has turned out to be a disaster').

Some strategies for challenging negative thoughts include:

- Specifying the situations that lead to stress. Not all situations are uniformly stressful.
- Questioning the evidence for a negative perception, and critically considering the probability of the negative perception being true.
- Checking whether expectations of oneself are unrealistic. Observing how other people handle similar situations.

3. Engineering and exposing oneself to achievable and pleasurable tasks can help to raise self-esteem and build self-confidence. If these tasks relate to other long-term goals, it is likely that their achievement will also engender a sense of mastery over other life events. Another strategy that may help to raise self-esteem is to document all achievements, however minor, or alternatively, to mention those achievements to others. Self-reward can be used to maintain new behaviours and to help acknowledge achievements.

4. Structured problem-solving (described in Chapter 12) is a strategy that will help to manage worries and break the cycle of ruminations that characterise this personality style. Structured problem-solving can be used in conjunction with cognitive challenges to refine and specify the types of worries and then to address those problems in a rational manner.

5. Goal-setting and time management are useful to limit the amount of time spent ruminating on perceived problems by harnessing that emotional energy and channelling it to more productive uses in achieving goals. Setting long- and short- term goals gives purpose to activities and helps the individual keep the broader picture 'in focus'.

An example of goal-setting

Where would you like to see yourself in 10 years time? What would you like your life to be like?

In your social life	Occupationally	Financially	Family relationships
Regular group of close friends	Own my own business	Own my home	Improve relationship with elder sister

What would you need to do in the next 12–18 months in order to achieve these goals?

In your social life	Occupationally	Financially	Family relationships
Start contacting old friends or cultivating new friends	Consider doing a small business course	Set up a savings plan	Start attending family functions

---

6. Learning to tolerate and manage uncomfortable emotions is an important skill that needs to be developed in order to improve self-reliance and

minimise excessive reassurance-seeking from others. This may involve acknowledging unpleasant emotions and learning to self-talk and self-soothe to reduce distress.

Building resilience

The natural propensity for people with this personality style is to ruminate over the outcome of actual or potential events. Such mulling over can be harnessed and productively channelled into effective problem-solving skills. Individuals with an anxious worrying personality style may be better able to brainstorm creative solutions to their problems once they learn how to look at the 'flip' side of negative or dysfunctional thoughts.

Barriers to effective intervention

Maladaptive features of such a temperament are probably long standing and will be difficult to change in the short term. It is possible that setbacks during the course of therapy may result in a reversion to old dysfunctional thinking and behavioural patterns. Encouragement for change may need to be given throughout the course of therapy in order to reinforce the acquisition of new skills.

The role of medication

Patients presenting with a non-melancholic depression and an anxious worrying personality style tend to achieve considerable benefit from the selective serotonin reuptake inhibitors (SSRIs). These mute the worrying and emotional dysregulation, allowing distance from perceived problems. Patients commonly report that the problems remain but they feel that, with an SSRI, they are 'swimming' rather than 'sinking'.

The SSRIs have the capacity to normalise worry. Too high a dose can render the patient 'blahed out' and not 'worried enough'. Some patients will need to stay on SSRIs for extended periods, others benefit from receiving such medicine for a period sufficient to re-set their own 'rheostat', while others benefit from a second phase of more focussed non-medication therapy (as detailed) and no longer need medication.

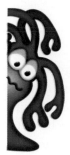

19

The social avoidance personality style and non-melancholic depression

Social avoidance personality style

People with features of this personality style tend to shy away from social stimulation and are usually reluctant to socialise or mix with others at parties or other social gatherings. They may appear shy or distant around people, especially those they have not previously met. Features of this personality style include a preference for solitude and solitary activities. There is the danger that, when stressed or upset, people with features of this type of personality style completely withdraw from social activity and thus hinder the likelihood of deriving support from others, including seeking professional help.

Key features of the Social Avoidant Personality Style (derived from our Temperament and Personality Questionnaire):
- Dislikes social stimulation or mixing with others.
- Avoids parties and other social gatherings.
- Reserved in social situations.
- Quiet around others.
- Holds back on meeting new people.
- Prefers own company to that of others.

High levels of anxiety and self-criticism in social situations may characterise this personality style. There may also be a history of early adverse experiences surrounding social situations, such as being bulled or humiliated at school or teased by siblings at home. People with features of this personality style may have organised their lives to exclude or minimise interaction with others. For example, by choosing occupations that require solitary rather than team activities, and maintaining a small group of friends and acquaintances who are unlikely to threaten or make demands on their time.

Under stress, such people are likely to withdraw into themselves, to actively avoid social contact and to engage in solitary activities that either distract from their distress or alleviate their mood. They may risk alienating those around them by not wanting to discuss their problems or by avoidance behaviours. Furthermore, their solitary pursuits exclude those who are able to offer assistance and help alleviate such distress.

Under stress the Social Avoidance Personality Style is characterised by:
- Withdrawal from others.
- Active avoidance of social situations.
- Pursuit of solitary activities.
- Exclusion of possible social supports.

The psychotransmitter model

Our neuronal model includes a saliency mechanism that scans for certain types of stressors and receptor hypersensitivity to specific types of psychotransmitters ('key and lock' model). Faulty ion channels (perceptual and attributional styles) which are hyper-responsive further encourage stimulation by specific types of psychotransmitters. Intracellular proteins and enzymes (defences, coping repertoires, and cognitive schemas) are overwhelmed by the level of neuronal stimulation (reinforcing cognitive schemas of inadequacy). Complex second messengers are produced which incorporate aspects of the stressor (e.g. feeling invalidated by others) and which switch off self-esteem resulting in a depressive reaction (Figs 19.1–19.4).

This model relies on the interplay of:
- Receptor hypersensitivity.
- Down-regulation to reduce the potential of 'aversive' stimulation.
- Faulty ion channels which are selective for particular types of ions (experiences).
- An interaction between those ions and intracellular mediators to effect the overall down-regulation of the 'neuron'.
- Processes that switch off self-esteem.

Treatment would need to address a number of issues including receptor hypersensitivity ('key and lock' model) and 'inoculation' to potentially aversive types of psychotransmitters. However, there would also be the need to correct faulty ion channels (perceptual and attributional styles) and address the interactions of those processes with intracellular mediators (coping repertoires and cognitive schemas).

Fig. 19.1 Saliency mechanism and receptor hyper-sensitivity to certain types of stressors.

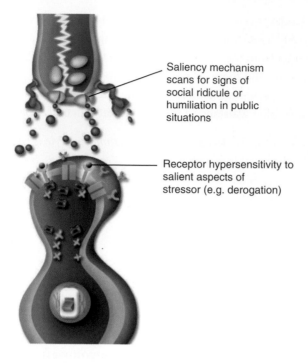

Saliency mechanism scans for signs of social ridicule or humiliation in public situations

Receptor hypersensitivity to salient aspects of stressor (e.g. derogation)

Fig. 19.2 Ion channels and protean defences.

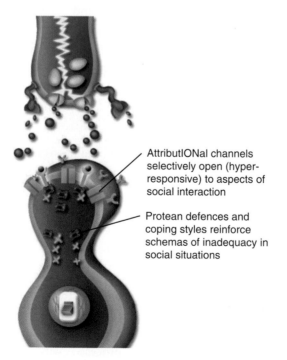

AttributIONal channels selectively open (hyper-responsive) to aspects of social interaction

Protean defences and coping styles reinforce schemas of inadequacy in social situations

The psychotransmitter model

Fig. 19.3 Production of second messengers incorporating some aspects of the stressor.

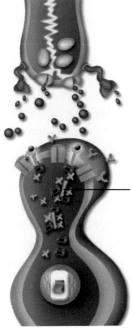

Production of second messengers incorporating prior adverse social interactions (e.g. feeling invalidated by others)

Fig. 19.4 Self-esteem switched off.

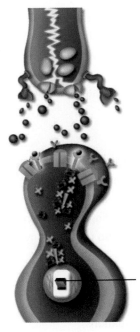

Self-esteem is switched off by second messengers

Case vignette – Alan

Alan is a 29-year old computer programmer who worked for a large multi-national corporation. Although he had worked for the company since he completed his university studies 6 years ago, he had not made any close friends. Instead, Alan preferred to spend his spare time in solitary activities such as reading or playing computer games. He had one close friend from his university days with whom he played regular tennis. Alan was well liked by his colleagues at work who considered him to be 'quiet' and was frequently invited to various work-related social functions. He usually declined such invitations but was experiencing increasing pressure from his managers to attend these and other social functions. Such pressure made him feel very stressed and he was beginning to feel tired all the time and was spending a lot of time sleeping. Following criticism from his manager about not being a 'team player', he became progressively depressed, isolating himself more and immersing himself in his computer games, and not playing tennis with his friend anymore.

Case summary

Alan's episode of depression is directly triggered by pressure from his managers to attend more company social functions. It is likely that many of his depressive symptoms would be significantly alleviated if this immediate pressure was removed. However, it is possible that Alan's socially isolated lifestyle increases the risk that he will encounter other social stressors needing to be addressed in the future. His increased level of social isolation in response to requests to attend work-related social functions will further exacerbate his anxieties about social situations in general and perpetuate his depressive episode.

Dysfunctional thoughts and attitudes

- Mixing with people makes me feel uncomfortable.
- Meeting new people makes me anxious.
- I do not like any changes to my social life.
- I know that others do not like spending time with me.
- I do not enjoy social situations as I do not have anything to talk about.

Summary of Alan's problem areas

- Poor social skills.
- High levels of anxiety in social situations.
- Restricted social contacts.

- Negative views about social interactions.
- A relatively inflexible lifestyle.

Principles of psychological intervention

Embarking on a course of psychological therapy is usually precipitated by involuntary and unavoidable lifestyle changes. People with personality features of social avoidance are likely to have built their lifestyles around the avoidance of social situations, as well as a pattern of routine and regular activities. When threatened by possible changes to their level of interaction with others they are likely to become distressed and try to restore previous lifestyle habits. Psychological treatment would need to address anxieties associated with immediate stressors, while providing exposure and instruction in coping with potential stressors in the future. Compared to the other personality styles described in this book, the socially avoidant personality style requires a strong focus on behavioural change in order to overcome a depressive illness and promote resilience to further episodes. Medium- to long-term intervention over a 6- to 12-month period is likely to be helpful. A strong therapeutic alliance based on trust is essential to effect change in social functioning.

In the short term, psychological strategies that alleviate high levels of anxiety in social situations are recommended. In the early stages of therapy, people with such personality features may prefer to engage in self-directed tasks which require minimal interaction with others, such as reading bibliotherapy books focusing on how to deal with social anxieties, or embarking on an exercise or meditation programme to reduce levels of autonomic arousal or anxiety. In the medium- to long-term, psychological interventions need to address the specific anxieties associated with the avoidance of social situations by examining and changing dysfunctional cognitions and behaviours in such situations. Group-based interventions involving others who share similar personality features can encourage exposure to social situations in a supportive environment.

A structure for psychological intervention
- Medium- to long-term therapy.
- Strong therapeutic alliance based on trust.
- Anxiety-reduction strategies.
- Address and change dysfunctional cognitions and behaviours associated with social situations.
- Group-based interventions may be useful.

What sort of therapist?

People with personality features of social avoidance may be difficult to engage in psychological therapy at the outset. Building an atmosphere of trust and reducing anticipatory anxiety concerning specific psychological strategies are essential before the commencement of therapy. Good rapport may be achieved by setting clear therapy goals and by an open and honest communication style in discussing the tasks and skills required to achieve those goals.

Getting started

A gentle non-confrontational approach to initiating therapy is required. This may include examination of current stressors and specific techniques for alleviating distress and addressing those concerns. Immediate relief from current stressors, if possible, will help build trust and strengthen rapport. Often, diagrammatic representation of the current difficulties, together with precipitating stressors and personal vulnerabilities, can help to provide a focus for psychological intervention. The joint development of such a diagram in the initial phases of therapy will also provide a reference point for later psychological improvements. A diagrammatic representation of current difficulties, precipitating factors, and personal vulnerabilities is illustrated in Fig. 19.5. This diagram can be referred to as therapy progresses in order to ensure that specific issues, that may otherwise be overlooked, are addressed.

Fig. 19.5 Developing a framework for therapy.

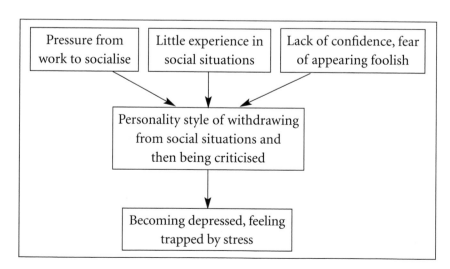

Written material about overcoming social anxieties or on improving self-confidence in social situations can provide discussion points about such issues at a personal level during therapy sessions. However, as therapy progresses, it would be necessary to focus less on written material and more on reviews of in vivo exposure to social situations as a focus of discussion.

Establishing the areas for intervention

Clear guidelines about the elements of therapeutic change will reduce the likelihood of excessive anxiety about the process and prevent the premature discontinuation of treatment. To this end it would be helpful to outline the key strategies that would be used to reduce current distress, control anxiety in social situations, and prevent the occurrence of further distress.

Problem area	Psychological intervention
• Distorted and negative thoughts about performance in social situations	• Question misconceptions and assumptions about social situations
• Social isolation from inadequate social support networks	• Reduce social isolation by actively expanding social support networks
• Lack of social competence in social situations due to lack of practice and/or lack of social skills	• Social skills training; role plays and modelling to learn more appropriate ways of behaving in social situations
• Possible low self-esteem and low sense of self-efficacy	• Graded exposure to positive social experiences
• Limited behavioural repertoires (e.g. avoiding social interaction when stressed)	• Anxiety-management strategies to control high levels of autonomic arousal in social situations

Intervention strategies

1. Questioning misconceptions and assumptions about social situations may be used to change dysfunctional thinking, especially about personal performance in social interactions. The therapist may commence challenging such dysfunctional thoughts right from the first session.
2. Expanding social support networks can serve several purposes. It provides exposure to a variety of social situations which would otherwise be

> ## Questioning misconceptions and assumptions
> *Assumptions*
> For example, *'I'm sure to dislike meeting my new neighbours'*
> *'Meeting new people is stressful. I never enjoy it'*
>
> The therapist's role in challenging such misconceptions might involve asking whether these feelings occur invariably or in all situations. Furthermore, the therapist could inquire how current friends and acquaintances were acquired if these assumptions were true in the past.
>
> Challenging these assumptions also serves to undermine other long-standing attitudes about social situations and introduce the possibility of changing thoughts and behaviours to reduce anxiety and distress.

avoided; it prevents social isolation by ensuring contact with a few social groups, thus bypassing possible problems in one of them; and it encourages the development of social supports in difficult times. Social support networks can develop by the individual joining interest or hobby groups, beginning a course of study, or participating in organised social functions.

3. Social skills training may include written material, behavioural modelling, and role plays of appropriate social skills by the therapist during therapy sessions. Videotaping behavioural exercises during therapy sessions can also provide a useful source of feedback to modify problems in social interaction.

4. Exposure to graded social events will help to desensitise to social situations, especially if a system of self-rewards is used to mark the successful completion of each task. The use of rewards, at least in the early phase of therapy, is not to be minimised or dismissed as it is important to build up a positive association with ongoing social interaction.

5. Anxiety-management strategies such as slow breathing and attention-focusing techniques can be used to ensure that anxiety does not escalate in social situations. Such techniques should be well learned before applying them in stressful social situations.

Building resilience

It is important to refer back to the initial problem formulation and assess whether some of the stressors have been modified or eliminated, and/or personal resilience to stressful situations has been increased. At the conclusion of therapy these changes may be documented in an amended diagram of current stressors and modified vulnerabilities.

Barriers to effective intervention

Social avoidance can re-surface during stressful periods which may be unrelated to the perceived stressfulness of actual social events. Instruction in stress-management strategies, such as relaxation and meditation techniques will help control overall levels of autonomic arousal.

The role of medication

Some of the newer antidepressants, including the selective serotonin reuptake inhibitors (SSRIs), are held to be useful and beneficial for those with social phobia (which overlaps with a personality style of social avoidance). In our experience, medication is generally less beneficial than the psychological interventional approach detailed here.

20

The personal reserve personality style and non-melancholic depression

Personal reserve personality style

Key features of this personality style include an apprehension about and a dislike of people getting too close at an emotional or personal level. People with this personality characteristic tend to pull away from closeness or intimacy and to hide their true feelings from others. They may also feel uneasy when others disclose their feelings or attempt to confide in them for emotional support. People with features of this personality style may derive pleasure from more superficial or casual social interactions and it is possible for them to have a wide circle of casual acquaintances with whom they interact on a regular basis. Such individuals, who are usually self-sufficient, resourceful and independent, often deny the need for more intense friendships or intimate attachments.

Key features of the Personal Reserve Personality Style (derived from our Temperament and Personality Questionnaire):
- Dislikes people getting too close at an emotional level.
- Withdraws from people when they get too close.
- Dislikes disclosing true feelings to others.
- Feels uncomfortable about others disclosing their feelings.
- Prefers to keep feelings to themselves.
- Does not seek advice from others.

Although such individuals normally engage in solitary activities, when stressed or upset they may completely withdraw from any social interaction and their tenuous friendships or fragile relationships may become strained with the risk of losing their already flimsy social support networks. Individuals with features of this personality style may never have learnt to interact with others at a personal level, to express their own fears and anxieties, or to actively ask for help when it is needed. Re-establishing social contacts after a period of stress or depression is especially difficult for such people and, in old age, they are likely to experience loneliness and feel marginalised among their peers. The risk of suicide may be higher for people with these personality features than with any of the other temperament or personality styles.

People with features of the personal reserve personality style are unlikely to confide in others when depressed. Thus, none of their friends or acquaintances may realise the extent of their distress or depression and then recommend professional help. If they seek psychological help, it will largely occur as a result of a realisation of the extent of their own problems, usually after several unsuccessful attempts at self-cure. In therapy, these individuals are likely to prematurely terminate treatment if they feel emotionally threatened by having to disclose too much of themselves too soon. Establishing good rapport at the outset of treatment can also pose challenges for the therapist.

Under stress the Personal Reserve Personality Style is characterised by:
- Withdrawal from any social interaction.
- Engagement in solitary activities.
- Feelings of loneliness.
- Inability to ask others for assistance.

The psychotransmitter model

Our neuronal model is similar to that of the social avoidant personality style (see Chapter 19) in that a saliency mechanism firstly scans the environment for certain types of stressors (e.g. criticism from others). Receptors are hypersensitive to certain types of psychotransmitters (especially those that convey a message of personal disclosure or intimacy) while attributIONal channels are selective to some types of ions (e.g. those that promote feelings of vulnerability). At the intracellular level, proteins and enzymes (defense mechanisms and dysfunctional cognitive schemas about personal disclosure or intimacy) reinforce feelings of vulnerability and threat. Second messengers incorporate aspects of the current stressor as well as prior adverse experiences of self-disclosure or intimacy and eventually switch off self-esteem resulting in depression (Figs 20.1–20.4).

This model relies on the interplay of:
- Receptor hypersensitivity.
- Ion channels which selectively open to some types of stimulation.
- Intracellular mediators which reinforce aversive aspects of stressor.
- Production of complex second messengers which switch off self-esteem.

Fig. 20.1 Saliency mechanism and receptor hyper-sensitivity to certain types of stressors.

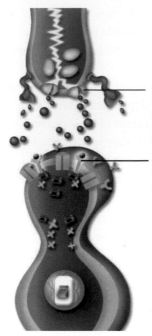

Saliency mechanism scans for criticism and other threats to self-esteem from significant others

Receptor hypersensitivity to salient aspects of stressor (e.g. feeling negatively judged or 'not measuring up' to significant other)

Fig. 20.2 AttributIONaL channels facilitate unpleasant feelings.

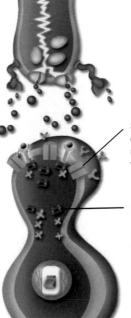

Selective attributIONal channels facilitate unpleasant feelings of vulnerability

Protean defences and coping styles reinforce schemas of vulnerability or threat

Fig. 20.3 Production
of second messengers
incorporating some
aspects of the
stressor.

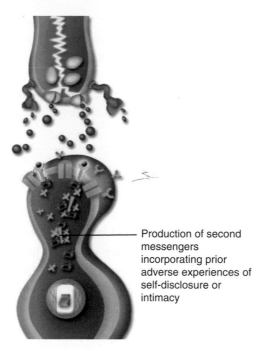

Production of second
messengers
incorporating prior
adverse experiences of
self-disclosure or
intimacy

Fig. 20.4 Self-esteem
is switched off.

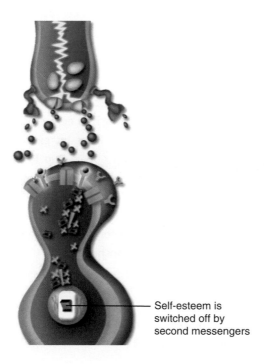

Self-esteem is
switched off by
second messengers

As with the social avoidant personality style psychotransmitter model, treatment would need to address a number of issues including receptor hypersensitivity ('key and lock' model) and 'inoculation' to potentially aversive types of psychotransmitters. This latter strategy may include graduated exposure to a range of aversive psychotransmitters (experiences involving personal disclosure and intimacy) at varying concentrations (different intensities of exposure).

Case vignette – Simon

Simon had always been described as a quiet person by his friends and workmates. At the age of 29, it had been 7 years since he graduated in engineering, with first class honours. Simon still kept up with his small university network of friends by playing regular sports and occasionally socialising with them on weekends. Although he enjoyed their company, he always felt somewhat uncomfortable with disclosing information about himself to his friends or when any of his friends tried to confide in him about their personal problems. Recently, he had met a young woman in whom he was beginning to take an interest. However, his discomfort with closeness and in revealing his intimate thoughts and feelings had prevented this relationship from developing further. She had told him on several occasions that she wondered whether he really cared for her and, once, in a fit of anger, had described him as a 'cold fish'. Simon was beginning to get depressed over the consequences of his reserve – he was losing her. He had withdrawn from contact with his friends and preferred to spend his time watching television alone in his flat.

Case summary

Simon's depression will worsen as he becomes progressively isolated from his friends and he has fewer outlets in which to derive enjoyment. He is more at risk of significant depression when he loses his girlfriend. Although he may recognise that he has problems with opening up to people, his feelings of intense discomfort and anxiety whenever he is confronted by potentially intimate interpersonal situations, and his lack of social skills prevent him from overcoming these problems. Therapy will need to focus on a combination of social skills training and strategies to overcome his unpleasant feelings when in potentially close and confiding relationships.

Dysfunctional thoughts and attitudes

- I cannot bear anyone to get too close to me.
- I am uneasy about others telling me personal things.

- I would rather handle my problems on my own.
- I am uncomfortable about sharing my feelings with others.
- No one could possibly know me well enough to help me.

Summary of Simon's problem areas

- Narrow opportunities to develop intimate or close relationships.
- Intense discomfort in close or intimate interpersonal situations.
- Lack of social skills to develop closer relationships.
- Coping skills (such as watching television or withdrawing from others) which perpetuate problems in the interpersonal area.

Principles of psychological intervention

People with features of this personality style usually require medium- to long-term psychological intervention in order to learn new interpersonal skills, overcome their anxieties about intimacy and closeness, and change dysfunctional or maladaptive habitual behaviours that distance them from others. Individual therapy sessions need to be highly structured with a clear focus on behavioural goals, at least in the early phases of treatment. In the middle to later phases of therapy, when the focus may be on attitudinal and behavioural change, sessions could be less structured, and emphasise trouble-shooting or problem-solving approaches.

Instruction in changing some key aspects of their lifestyle is probably necessary in order to prevent further depressive episodes. A key feature of therapy will be in working with the client to uncover lifestyle problems, such as the restriction of social activities to large impersonal gatherings, or avoiding novel experiences that may predispose towards loneliness and isolation in the long term. Setbacks during the course of therapy will need to be addressed immediately, as they can inadvertently reinforce long-established negative perceptions about modifying or changing behaviours.

A structure for psychological intervention
- Medium- to long-term therapy.
- Focus on learning interpersonal skills.
- Anxiety management about intimacy and closeness.
- Changing dysfunctional or maladaptive behaviours.
- Clear behavioural goals.
- Focus on changing dysfunctional aspects of lifestyle.

What sort of therapist?

A non-threatening, non-confrontational style is best in the early phases of treatment to prevent premature termination of therapy by the client. Building good rapport with the client will be a key therapeutic ingredient, not only to effect change but also in order to demonstrate and practise skills involved in controlling anxieties associated with self-disclosure. Once rapport has been established, a more confrontational approach may be used, if necessary. However, the therapist should bear in mind that excessive levels of anxiety during therapy can reinforce negative attitudes about disclosing intimate thoughts and feelings to others.

Getting started

People with personal reserve characteristics are likely to get distressed as a response to problems associated with or restrictions imposed by their lifestyles. They are likely to seek professional help when their routine is disrupted by events usually beyond their control, and only after they have exhausted self-help options. Generally independent and self-sufficient, they will seek help reluctantly. Their resourcefulness and previous attempts at overcoming their difficulties need to be acknowledged before a treatment plan can be jointly developed.

Next, clear behavioural goals should be jointly established by the client and therapist. These behavioural goals, which will help direct and shape the course of therapy, also provide a focus without eliciting excessive anxieties about self-disclosure in the early phase of treatment. The therapist needs to establish general goals which can be divided into a series of specific behavioural goals with clear indicators for their successful completion.

Setting behavioural goals for therapy

General goals	Specific goals	Indication of achievement
Not feeling lonely at home	Need to meet more people	Having the choice to talk to others
	Need to attend more social events	if lonely
Involved in a relationship	Need to ask someone out	Dating someone on a regular basis
	Need to be able to express feelings to others to establish a relationship	

Modification of these therapy goals may occur as new issues present themselves or existing goals are changed to accommodate recent insights or barriers to change.

Establishing the areas for intervention

There are many problem areas that will require attention during the course of therapy. Many can be addressed simultaneously while focusing on specific behavioural goals described in the previous section. It may be useful to forewarn the client of possible setbacks which may tempt them to revert to old, familiar but maladaptive ways of relating and behaving during the course of therapy.

Problem area	Psychological intervention
• Interpersonal skills deficits	• Social skills training
• Anxiety about intimacy, closeness and self-disclosure	• Anxiety-reduction strategies, desensitisation to self-disclosure, focus on early learning experiences
• Changing dysfunctional or maladaptive behaviours	• Role plays and behavioural modelling
• Focus on changing some aspects of lifestyle	• Problem-solving strategies, goal setting
• Narrow and fragile social network	• Improving social support networks, help develop an interest in others

Intervention strategies

1. Social skills training may be conducted in a group or individual approach. Social skills training may include learning specific skills in active listening, learning to make requests of others and knowing when to disclose personal information to others. A combination of didactic learning, active role play and in vivo practice is recommended.

2. A number of immediate anxiety-reduction strategies may be useful, such as slow breathing and attention re-focusing training. These strategies need to be used while engaging in moderately stressful activities related to personal self-disclosure or listening to others discussing their personal issues.

    Sometimes it is useful to explore early learning experiences which may have contributed to the development of these personality characteristics. Exploration of these issues would, however, only be relevant in cases where barriers to change are dependent upon understanding how the problem developed at an early age, and whether such information can be used to challenge current maladaptive cognitive and behavioural patterns.

3. Changing dysfunctional and maladaptive behaviour patterns may be achieved by role plays and modelling of more appropriate and adaptive behaviours in therapy sessions. Videotaping role plays followed by watching and requesting that the client comments on his or her problem behaviours can effect significant behavioural changes.

4. Problem-solving goal-setting strategies could be used to change aspects of lifestyle that could perpetuate dysfunctional ways of relating to others. Strategies could include browsing through magazines and newspapers for interesting social or educational events to relate to others.

5. Developing an interest in relating to others at a deeper level will need encouragement in the early stages by ensuring that there are rewards to be gained. This aspect may initially need to be reinforced with rewards that are not related to social interaction. Later, when intimate social interaction becomes a pleasurable activity in itself, those rewards can be phased out.

Building resilience

Maintaining a sense of 'connectedness' with others is likely to be a key issue in preventing relapse and in building resilience to future difficulties. It may be necessary to implement a plan for ensuring that the old habits of high levels of interpersonal reserve do not creep back. One method may be to engage in travelling or holidaying with friends on a regular basis where intimate bonds of friendship have a greater chance of being developed and maintained over time.

Barriers to effective intervention

There is always a high possibility of treatment attrition amongst people with personality features of personal reserve. Such individuals are often difficult to engage in therapy and are likely to be discouraged by any setbacks in their treatment. They may feel humiliated or embarrassed by failures on their part to engage others at a deeper emotional level. Reassurance and encouragement by the therapist throughout the process of therapy is necessary to ensure that they comply and continue with the proposed plan for recovery.

The role of medication

We are not persuaded that antidepressant medication is of distinct benefit for those who have this personality style as a dominant characteristic, and believe that psychosocial interventions are likely to be superior.

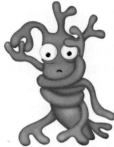

21

The rejection sensitivity personality style and non-melancholic depression

Rejection sensitivity personality style

This personality style is characterised by a tendency to worry about being rejected or abandoned by others. Key characteristics include being acutely tuned in to others' emotional needs and prone to feeling rejected. People with features of this personality style also tend to base their self-worth on others' perceptions of them and worry about the quality of their relationships with others. Although they may recognise that they tend to 'lose themselves' in relationships and become too attached, they are generally unable to prevent such pathological types of attachments from forming. As a direct result of their fears of abandonment, people with characteristics of the rejection sensitivity personality style may act in ways to please others at the expense of their own emotional health. Often, they may engage in and persist with abusive or dangerous relationships with others rather than leave the relationship altogether.

Key features of the Rejection Sensitivity Personality Style (derived from our Temperament and Personality Questionnaire):
- Worries about the quality of their relationships.
- Worries about being rejected or abandoned by others.
- Fears that their relationships may end.
- Feels as if their emotions are not reciprocated in relationships.
- Worries about what others think.
- Distressed about being alone.

When they experience difficulties in their relationships, such individuals may report feelings of intense emptiness and despair. Often the problems they describe in their relationships may be magnified to such an extent as to appear insurmountable. When upset over their relationships, people with features of this personality style may actively seek others for reassurance and support. However, their distress may be heightened if reassurance is not forthcoming or easily available. Characteristics when distressed may also include a tendency to engage in a variety of self-consoling behaviours such as spending more money, sleeping more, overeating/or bingeing on comfort foods. Loneliness, tiredness, mood swings and reactivity to minor stresses are also key features especially when distressed. Other 'atypical depression features' include hypersomnia and extreme fatigue (sometimes described as 'leaden paralysis').

People with characteristics of the rejection sensitivity personality style are more likely to seek help, compared to those with features of the other personality styles. Although people with heightened rejection sensitivity are likely to be compliant with therapy, there is the risk of dependency on the therapist, so that the appropriate termination of therapy can present difficult challenges.

Under stress the Rejection Sensitivity Personality Style is characterised by:
• Hypersomnolence.
• Hyperphagia for comfort foods.
• Ruminations about feelings of abandonment.
• Over-dependence on others.

The psychotransmitter model

This model involves hypersensitivity to and over-stimulation from specific types of psychotransmitters, together with a filtering mechanism which selects and responds to certain types of stimulation. Our model starts with problems of receptor hypersensitivity to specific types of psychotransmitters (especially those related to interpersonal conflict). Highly selective ion channels help to filter the way in which psychotransmitter are interpreted (e.g. personalising the stressor) and augment the level of aversive stimulation within the neuron (Figs 21.1 and 21.2).

Intracellular proteins (immature defenses and poor coping responses) and enzymes (cognitive schemas) fail to neutralise the aversive stimulation. Complex second messengers (encrusted with perceptions of abandonment and loss) switch off self-esteem resulting in depression (Figs 21.3 and 21.4).

This model relies on the interplay of:
• Receptor hypersensitivity.
• Highly selective ion channels.
• Ineffective intracellular proteins and enzymes.
• Processes that switch off self-esteem.

Intervention strategies may need to focus on reducing the overall excitability of the neuron, especially with respect to specific types of psychotransmitters,

Fig. 21.1 Receptor
hypersensitivity to
salient aspects of the
stressor.

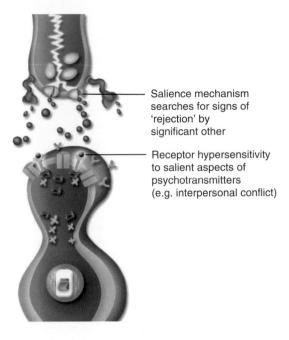

Salience mechanism
searches for signs of
'rejection' by
significant other

Receptor hypersensitivity
to salient aspects of
psychotransmitters
(e.g. interpersonal conflict)

Fig. 21.2
AttributIONal
channels personalise
the stressor.

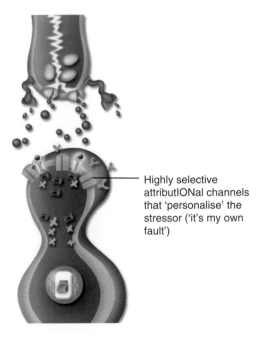

Highly selective
attributIONal channels
that 'personalise' the
stressor ('it's my own
fault')

gradually decreasing the level of stimulation to lower the resting 'set-point'. Intracellular processes (immature defenses, poor coping styles and dys-functional cognitive schemas) which affect the quality of second messenger psychotransmitters may also need to be directly addressed and corrected.

Fig. 21.3 Immature
defences and coping
repertoires.

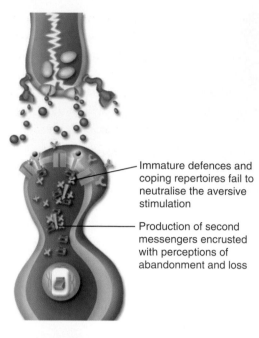

Immature defences and
coping repertoires fail to
neutralise the aversive
stimulation

Production of second
messengers encrusted
with perceptions of
abandonment and loss

Fig. 21.4 Second
messengers switch
off self-esteem.

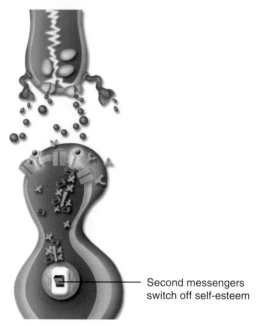

Second messengers
switch off self-esteem

Case vignette – Claire

Claire, a 33-year-old secretary, agonised over every perceived slight by her
boyfriend, Sam, and her girlfriends. After a night out with Sam, Claire would
usually return home feeling anxious and uncomfortable. She would suffer from

frequent bouts of extreme distress, accompanied by panic attacks, wondering whether her boyfriend really loved her or her friends cared for her as much as she for them. Claire would worry about the quality of her relationships and feared being abandoned by Sam or her friends. She allowed her friends to take advantage of her by lending them money and offering to drive them around. Over time, her friends became tired of her constant need for reassurance and would sometimes exclude her from their social activities. If Claire found out that she had been left out of these social events, she would plunge into a deep depression fuelled by feelings of inadequacy and worthlessness. She would experience feelings of 'emptiness' and loss, and become highly reactive to minor stresses.

In order to alleviate her mood, she would seek reassurance of friendship and support from her acquaintances. She would also engage in a variety of self-consoling and comforting behaviours such as bingeing on comfort foods, or indulging in warm baths, spending more money on clothes and grooming products, and oversleeping.

Case summary

Claire's insecurity about relationships has resulted in behaviours which have ultimately strained or eroded others' attachments to her. Her friends sometimes get exasperated and exclude her from their activities, which reinforces her negative attitudes and perceptions about abandonment and desirability as a friend or romantic partner. She indulges in self-consoling and escapist behaviours when distressed, but these will not resolve her relationship difficulties in the long term.

Dysfunctional thoughts and attitudes

- I cannot survive on my own.
- I need others to support me and reassure me.
- People will leave me if I do not please them.
- Who I am is determined by what others think of me.

Summary of Claire's problem areas

- Self-image based on others' perceptions.
- Worries about the quality of her relationships.
- Loses sense of 'self' when around significant others.
- Lack of assertiveness due to insecurity.
- Behaviours which perpetuate feelings of low self-worth and insecurity.

Principles of psychological intervention

Psychological intervention for individuals with these personality features needs to focus on interpersonal issues at the outset perhaps by even using the therapeutic relationship as a model for change. For example, the quality of the ongoing relationship with the therapist may be used to challenge long-standing dysfunctional thoughts and behaviours towards others. Medium- to long-term therapy is recommended during which sensitivity to abandonment or possible rejection by others is the focus of treatment. Clear goals for therapy and a proposed therapy termination date should also be established at the outset in order to prevent or lessen the development of excessive dependency on the therapist.

During the course of therapy, it is likely that behavioural changes toward others will affect the quality of those relationships. These relationship shifts can engender heightened levels of anxiety, feelings of abandonment, and insecurity. It may therefore be necessary to involve partners, family, and friends in the therapy process so that such changes can be discussed and understood by others. It may also be necessary to confront and challenge the extent of support and reassurance given by significant others as this may perpetuate excessive dependency.

A structure for psychological intervention

- Medium- to long-term therapy.
- Focus on interpersonal issues at the outset.
- Use the therapeutic relationship as a model for change.
- Clear goals and possible therapy termination date determined at the outset.
- Include significant others in the therapy process.

What sort of therapist?

People with features of the rejection sensitivity personality style are likely to quickly develop a close and trusting relationship with their therapist. A therapist who is empathic and supportive but who can also set firm limits and enforce therapy goals would be most effective. As the therapeutic relationship develops, the relationship itself may be used to challenge and change dysfunctional thoughts and behaviours in other situations. However, the therapist has to be mindful of dependency developing within the therapeutic relationship and attempt to maintain strict control over interpersonal and professional boundaries.

Getting started

People with features of this personality style are likely to seek treatment because of real or imagined problems in their relationships. Often they may report feelings of helplessness or ineffectiveness in their dealings with others, particularly close friends and romantic partners. Formulating a treatment plan may be best accomplished by using a narrative approach in order to help the patient understand how long-standing attitudes and behaviours may have shaped some of their significant life experiences and contributed to their current difficulties. Narrative approaches can also be used to draw on previously empowering experiences in which the individual managed to overcome their anxieties associated with rejection sensitivity and interpersonal stressors.

Developing a framework for therapy

Using a narrative approach, the therapist listens to how problems are described as 'stories' by the patient. For sensitivity to rejection personality features, the therapist may help the patient consider how certain attitudes and behaviours may have contributed to specific life choices.

For example, a therapist may ask 'Could it be that this event resulted from a choice based on long-standing attitudes or thoughts rather than simply by accident?' and suggest alternative outcomes to previous life events if different choices were made.

Encouraging the patient to document these life stories and the meanings they extracted from those experiences could also provide insights into problem areas.

The first exercise should help to highlight the key problem areas that require intervention in both the short- and the long term. It will also help to focus attention during the therapy sessions on early life experiences which may have contributed to the development of a high level of sensitivity to interpersonal issues. Recognition of early conflicts or threats of abandonment at an early stage of life may form the basis of therapeutic role plays or behavioural modelling exercises during the course of therapy.

An empowering exercise based on a narrative approach may be used to conclude the session. In this exercise, the patient may describe a number of situations in which they did not let their negative emotions and irrational thoughts get the better of them. The therapist may then draw from these experiences specific strategies that the patient used to overcome their anxieties in those situations that can be used in other similar situations in the future.

Establishing the areas for intervention

Establishment of therapy goals, rules, and personal boundaries are important during the early stages of therapy. People with such sensitivity to rejection are usually acutely aware of subtle nuances in their therapists' speech or manner that support their negative perceptions about interpersonal issues. At the outset it may be helpful to encourage open discussion and clarification of any interpersonal misperceptions occurring during the early stages of therapy. It may also be useful to prepare the patient for the possibility that, with their sanction, significant others such as close friends or partners may be invited to attend one or more sessions.

Problem area	Psychological intervention
• Feelings of helplessness and power-lessness in relationships	• Assertiveness training, role plays and behavioural modelling
• Distorted cognitive schemas about rejection and abandonment by others	• Cognitive challenges of dysfunctional thoughts and behavioural 'experiments'
• Vulnerability to tolerating rather than resolving interpersonal difficulties	• Expanding social networks and assertiveness training
• Loss of sense of 'self' in relationships	• Positive affirmations, improve self-esteem, and confidence
• High levels of anxiety	• Anxiety-reduction strategies, distraction techniques
• Lack of skills in resolving inter-personal problems or disputes	• Assertiveness training, role plays, and behavioural modelling

Intervention strategies

1. Assertiveness training, role plays, and behavioural modelling can be used to assist in problem areas such as overcoming feelings of helplessness and powerlessness in relationships, dealing with abusive or dysfunctional relationships and in gaining skills in resolving interpersonal disputes. This involves learning and practising adaptive phrases and non-verbal behaviours that may be used as required in real situations. It is best learnt in a step-wise manner beginning with some key assertive phrases such as 'I am not satisfied with ...., I would prefer it if you would do ...'. Role plays may be used to demonstrate the impact of certain behaviours on others during therapy sessions while behavioural modelling of more adaptive behaviours may be practised in vivo.

2. Cognitive challenges may be used to modify distorted thoughts about fears of abandonment or rejection by others. Using a structured step-wise approach, it is possible to critically examine these negative self-statements and challenge the 'supporting' evidence.

Identifying and challenging negative self-statements

In the first column, identify the negative self-statements about abandonment or rejection by others. In the second column, list the sources of 'evidence' for that negative self-statement

Negative self-statement	Evidence for negative self-statement
For example, '*My boyfriend wants to break up with me*'	'*He was quiet tonight*' '*He seemed preoccupied*'

Next, critically examine the self-statements and consider whether they truly provide evidence for the negative self-statement. Could there be another explanation for those behaviours? How may the same behaviours be re-interpreted?

Other explanations for behaviours	Re-interpreting that behaviour
'*He may have had other issues on his mind*' '*He may have wanted to spend time thinking about something urgent*'	'*He was probably quiet because of these other issues and not because he wants to break off our relationship*'

Behavioural 'experiments' may be used to test the premises underlying such thoughts. For example, a number of behavioural tasks could be developed to test whether assertive behaviours result in abandonment or rejection by others. At the completion of each activity, it would be useful to ask how the task has changed any negative self-perceptions.

3. There are numerous practical ways in which social networks can be broadened. For example, joining hobby or sports clubs, enrolling in short courses of study, or attending organised social functions. The aim of expanding social networks is twofold: firstly, it is to provide enjoyment in social interactions with others especially when primary relationships may be stressful or hurtful. Secondly, benefits may be gained by learning about how others relate well to the people around them.

4. Practising positive affirmations, improving self-esteem, and self-confidence may be achieved by engaging in activities that result in a sense of achievement or accomplishment. A list of tasks based on short- and long-term goals can help structure activities over a period of time.

5. When stressed by perceived interpersonal difficulties, individuals with features of the rejection sensitivity personality style may suffer from heightened levels of anxiety which will be ameliorated, to some extent, by

reassurance from others. To modify this maladaptive behaviour, it is necessary to consider techniques that will reduce anxiety such as progressive muscle relaxation, breathing exercises, and meditative techniques. Distraction techniques, described in previous chapters, may also be used to prevent repetitive seeking of reassurance from others.

Building resilience

The key vulnerabilities to depression in this personality style are feelings of rejection, abandonment and loss, together with a lack of individual identity (demonstrated by a sense of 'merging' with others). In the long term, in order to build resilience, it would be necessary to help strengthen that sense of self and self-worth independently of their relationships with others. This may be achieved by helping them acknowledge and own, among other things, their strengths and weaknesses, needs and desires, and successes and failures, as a means of clarifying their individual identity.

Barriers to effective intervention

Pathological styles of relating that develop over long periods of time are difficult to change in the short term and it is easy for patients to become demoralised by setbacks. Furthermore, others' behaviours and styles of relating to the patient may need to be directly addressed despite positive changes being made by the depressed patient. Being mindful of these possible problem areas will help prevent resistance or premature termination of psychological therapy.

The role of medication

Monoamine oxidase inhibitor (MAOI) medication has long been held to have specific benefits for the 'atypical depression' contributed to strongly by such a personality style. While it may be helpful, its side-effects and the need for care in prescription and management argue against it being viewed as a first-line drug treatment. We find selective serotonin reuptake inhibitor (SSRI) antidepressants to be equally helpful to many such patients – particularly when they have panic attacks and other features suggesting high trait anxiety. Generally, medication needs to be combined with psychological interventions (as illustrated above) to achieve the best results.

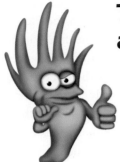

22

The self-focused personality style and non-melancholic depression

Self-focused personality style

Key features of this type of personality style are a lack of consideration or tolerance for others' needs. The individual's low frustration tolerance may be related to failure, relating to their early developmental experiences, to learn how to delay immediate gratification. People who have features of this personality style may display a tendency to blame others to make sense of their feelings of distress when things go wrong, rather than shouldering blame themselves. Others may find people with these personality features unhelpful or unempathic towards them, especially at times when they require assistance. People with this personality style tend to take advantage of others' limitations and shortcomings. They may behave in ways that suggest a sense of entitlement or privilege at the expense of others' comfort or welfare, and may inappropriately disregard others when pursuing their own goals. When depressed they may become quite 'hostile' and provocative to those around, often having a hair trigger explosive response to having their needs frustrated.

Key features of the Self-focused Personality Style (derived from our Temperament and Personality Questionnaire):
- Do not put themselves out for anyone.
- Intolerant of others' wishes.
- Unsympathetic to others.
- Take advantage of others.
- Enjoy manipulating people.
- Blame others when things go wrong.
- Often hostile and volatile in their interactions with others.

When distressed, people with features of this personality style commonly engage in risk-taking behaviours such as excessive drinking, smoking, or gambling. Key characteristics when stressed also include anger toward others when their needs or wants are thwarted. At the extreme end of the spectrum, such people may physically lash out, destroy property or cause physical harm to those around them. Such individuals may surround themselves with those that are emotionally dependent or needy. In the long term, individuals displaying strong self-focused personality characteristics are likely to be lonely and socially isolated. They are likely to suffer from episodes of depression if their needs are repeatedly unmet and/or if they lose their network of 'useful' friends and acquaintances. They are also likely to experience episodes of depression when frustrated from achieving their goals by others.

When they seek help, it is usually because of a life crisis such as debts, being charged with assault, or being evicted from their home because of violent or abusive behaviour. It is unlikely that they will recognise how their own behaviours may have contributed to their current crisis. Instead, they may try to shift the blame for their difficulties onto their friends and acquaintances and strongly believe that their difficulties can only be resolved by changes in others' behaviours. Individuals with features of this personality style pose considerable challenges in therapy as they may not choose to assume responsibility for alleviating their own distress.

Under stress the Self-focused Personality Style is characterised by:
• Engaging in risk-taking behaviours.
• Self-serving behaviours.
• Low frustration tolerance.
• Anger and hostility directed against others.

The psychotransmitter model

The self-focused personality style is characterised by a sense of entitlement, self-gratifying behaviours and a lowered threshold for frustration tolerance. This process lends itself to a model in which receptors are sensitive only to certain types of stimulation (particularly those that obstruct goal-attainment). Partially open ion channels (perceptual and attributional styles that tend to blame others) are over-restrictive in monitoring the passage of substances into the neuron while ineffective intracellular proteins and enzymes (immature defenses and coping repertoires) are unable to modulate the level of excitation in the neuron. Over time, the neuron becomes over-stimulated resulting in energy surges (angry outbursts) which disrupt its functioning (failure to achieve goals). Second messengers become modified by neuronal dysregulation (encrusted with a sense of powerlessness) which switch off self-esteem (Figs 22.1–22.4).

The psychotransmitter model

Fig. 22.1 Receptor hypersensitivity and restrictive ion channels.

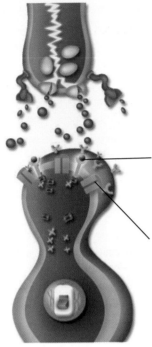

Receptor hypersensitivity 'flares up' in response to certain stressors (e.g. not getting one's own way)

Partially open attributIONal channels (focus on blaming others to maintain self-esteem)

Fig. 22.2 Limited defences and coping repertoires.

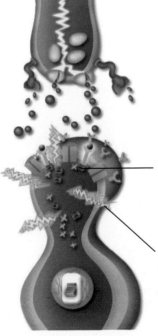

Limited defences and coping repertoires (insight) for modulating emotional reactions

Neuron becomes over-stimulated resulting in energy surges (angry outbursts)

Fig. 22.3 Second messengers reflect a sense of powerlessness.

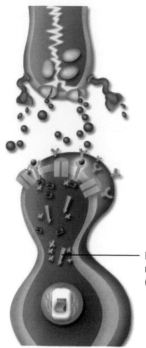

Failure to achieve goals modifies second messengers (sense of powerlessness)

Fig. 22.4 Second messengers switch off self-esteem.

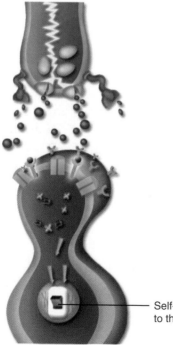

Self-esteem switches to the off position

This model relies on the interplay of:

- Receptor hypersensitivity to certain types of psychotransmitters.
- Restrictive ion channels.
- Defective intracellular proteins and enzymes.
- Second messengers which switch off self-esteem.

Immediate treatment strategies would have to decrease sensitivity to certain types of stimulation (life events and life stressors) and increase the level of stimulation (and enjoyment) from other more appropriate sources. In the long term, other problems associated with receptor site binding ('key and lock' model, interpretations, and reactions to certain types of life events particularly those that obstruct goal attainment) and faulty ion channels (perceptual and attributional biases that tend to blame others) may need to be addressed in order to prevent relapse.

Case vignette – Matthew

Others had always found Matthew impatient and dismissive in his dealings with them. Matthew himself was intolerant of other people, especially when he felt that they stood between him and his wishes. In his interactions with others, he often demonstrated a disparaging or condescending attitude and a lack of consideration or tolerance for their needs. He displayed a tendency to blame others to make sense of his feelings of distress when things went wrong. His friends and acquaintances tolerated his dismissive attitude but considered him unhelpful and uncaring towards them.

When distressed, which usually occurred when events did not work out to his advantage, Matthew would indulge in drinking binges, chain smoke, or lose money gambling on the poker machines at the local club. When extremely upset, Matthew would physically lash out at others and damage or destroy property such as furniture, household ornaments, and punch holes in walls and doors. After one of these outbursts, Matthew would often blame others around him for provoking him into an uncontrollable rage. Depression would generally follow brief moments of insight when he would be aware of his powerlessness and failure to achieve his primary goals.

Case summary

The likelihood of Matthew becoming depressed for other than brief periods is possibly lower than for most of the other personality styles. He displays only partial insight into his own behaviour and blames others for his own behavioural problems, so that his self-esteem is less vulnerable to dropping. However, when his plans are thwarted by events beyond his control, Matthew is likely to become distressed and engage in maladaptive coping behaviours, many of which are solitary and self-destructive pursuits, and which are likely to exacerbate the impact of current stressors and worsen his mood.

Dysfunctional thoughts and attitudes

- My needs are more important that anyone else's.
- Other people should acquiesce to my needs and desires.
- It is other people's fault that I get angry.
- It is usually other people's fault when things go wrong.
- Other people should change so that they do not upset me.

Summary of Matthew's problem areas

- Poor tolerance of frustrations and setbacks.
- Lack of responsibility for his feelings and behaviours.
- Poor communication skills.
- Few social supports and limited social support network.
- Coping styles that are likely to exacerbate his problems.

Principles of psychological intervention

People with features of the self-focused personality style are less likely to seek professional help than those with features of the other personality styles. Treatment may be sought as a last resort, usually to salvage a deteriorating interpersonal situation or to avoid punishment by the law. Structured short-term psychological intervention with a focus on specific strategies for behavioural change in the short term, such as problem-solving approaches, may be useful.

One aim of therapy is to help break the spiral of self-destructive behaviours which will ultimately worsen distress and exacerbate a depressive episode. Destructive behaviours, such as gambling or drinking to excess, will worsen the impact of current stressors and create additional problems which also have to be addressed. It is necessary, as a first step, to curtail or diminish the impact of these secondary behaviours. Once these behaviours are controlled, then it may be possible to address some of the underlying problems associated with this personality style.

Unless willing to accept that their problems are largely attributable to their dysfunctional attitudes and style of relating to others, people who have these personality features are unlikely to seek change. Nevertheless, it would be helpful to provide information on respecting others' rights and property, teach them effective communication skills (conflict resolution and anger management) and help them reflect on the long term adverse consequences of their dysfunctional behaviours.

A structure for psychological intervention

- Structured short-term therapy.
- Focus on specific strategies for behavioural change.
- Break spiral of self-destructive behaviours.
- Conflict resolution and anger management.
- Information on respecting others' rights and property and facilitate reflection on long-term adverse consequences of their dysfunctional behaviours.

What sort of therapist?

People with self-focused personality features will relate best to a therapist who is able to offer support, while setting firm expectations and limits especially on inappropriate or violent behaviours within or outside therapy sessions and manipulative behaviours during the course of therapy. The therapist also needs to be mindful of other processes during the course of therapy which may wrest control of the sessions from the therapist or sabotage the process of therapy. Premature discontinuation of therapy is always a high probability among individuals with these personality features, especially when improvements in mood are perceived to be too slow or when their sense of entitlement is perceived as not being respected by the therapist.

Getting started

Formulation of the presenting problems should be brief and heavily focused on current stressors and difficulties. Setting firm boundaries for inappropriate behaviours should also be addressed at the outset. Once the formulation of the presenting problem has been conducted, beginning with secondary behavioural problems (which usually are responsible for eliciting the most distress) can be a useful way to engage the client and commence the therapeutic process.

Establishing the areas for intervention

Once a problem formulation has been developed and presented to the patient, it becomes easier to decide on, by mutual consent, the key targets for intervention. In presenting the problem formulation, it may still be necessary to prioritise the order in which problems are to be addressed.

Problem area	Psychological intervention
• Poor tolerance of frustrations and setbacks	• Strategies to diffuse high levels of arousal
• Poor communication skills	• Assertiveness training, social skills training, conflict resolution skills
• Few social supports and limited social support networks	• Engagement in social groups with similar interests
• Coping styles that are likely to exacerbate existing problems	• Alternate strategies to coping with stressful situations
• Anger and hostility	• Anger management

Intervention strategies

1. High levels of arousal may manifest in aberrant or destructive behaviours aimed at dissipating the discomfort. Alternate strategies such as 'time out' or distraction techniques may be taught to alleviate heightened and aversive levels of arousal. It is unlikely that meditation techniques would be particularly helpful as they would demand a degree of concentration and discipline that may be difficult.

2. Assertiveness training and social skills training will help address deficits in communication style that lead to interpersonal problems. Role plays and behavioural modelling during therapy sessions can provide practical guidance for changing dysfunctional behaviours. Furthermore, the therapeutic relationship may be used as a working model for changing dysfunctional interpersonal behaviours and teaching skills in conflict resolution.

3. Encouraging participation in social groups with similar interests may provide a useful outlet for managing negative emotional states such as aggression or frustration. For example, sports such as boxing or wrestling may provide a socially acceptable outlet for pent-up emotions. Joining social groups would also possibly help expand social networks and provide a forum for practising recently acquired social skills.

4. Self-destructive behaviours, such as excessive gambling or drinking which help to reduce feelings of dysphoria, may be curbed by the use of aversive conditioning techniques such as covert sensitisation. Such strategies lessen the likelihood that these behaviours will promote relief from dysphoric feelings, and thus help to extinguish maladaptive and self-destructive behaviours. The use of aversive conditioning would need to be paired

with the provision and encouragement of other more adaptive coping skills, such as engaging in vigorous physical activity or participating in group social activities.

5. Anger management techniques can help to correct and replace previous dysfunctional behaviours relating to the expression of anger and frustration. Anger management encompasses a number of related techniques which help identify specific events that trigger angry reactions, common ways of reacting to anger and frustration, and methods by which such responses can be curbed or modified.

Building resilience

Building resilience to future depressive episodes for this personality style involves learning to tolerate frustration and curb impulsivity. It may also be helpful to engage in regular self-reflective strategies (e.g. discussing or writing about the impact of one's behaviours on others or considering how previous events may have unfolded if one had behaved in a different way). Resilience can also be fostered by peer-group membership, especially where there is a strong sense of leadership and purpose together with a clear and enforceable code of conduct for its members (e.g. Police Boys Club).

Barriers to effective intervention

Premature termination of treatment is likely to occur if change is perceived to be too slow, unrewarding, or too demanding in the short term. Treatment attrition can be prevented by frequent progress reviews. Once begun, therapy can be derailed by more pressing lifestyle stressors that may require immediate resolution. Nevertheless, it is important for the therapist to maintain control of sessions and direct the course of interventions using possible interruptions and distractions as an opportunity to practise new skills.

The role of medication

Studies (e.g. Blashfield & Morey, 1979) have examined and largely rejected the usefulness of both antidepressant and antipsychotic drugs in depressed patients with such a personality style. Medication is therefore unlikely to be helpful again because people with this personality style generally experience brief episodes, and as it can be used in a suicidal attempt when new episodes of depression commence.

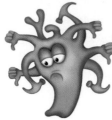

23

The self-critical personality style and non-melancholic depression

Self-critical personality style

People who display features of this personality style have an enduring tendency to blame themselves when anything goes wrong. They also tend to be self-critical and demanding on themselves to an irrational extent. Although they may prefer it when others take control of tasks, they are still likely to berate themselves for one or another aspect of the job. People with features of the self-critical personality style do not expect the high level of perfection that perfectionists demand of themselves and of others. Rather, they are more likely to believe that others will perform much better than they would at the same tasks. They may regularly seek reassurance from others about their own performance but such reassurance may be short-lived or only last until the next task. They often have a developmental history of uncaring and/or abusive parenting and other deprivational experiences.

Key features of the Self-critical Personality Style (derived from our Temperament and Personality Questionnaire):
- Tendency to be extremely tough on themselves.
- Extremely self-critical.
- Difficulty in measuring up to own standards.
- Prefers others to take control and make decisions.
- Others say they are too hard on themselves.
- Reliance on others for praise and reassurance.

Under stress, people who display features of this personality style are likely to become indecisive and lose focus on their immediate goals. Reassurance from others may assuage some anxieties in the short term but the same insecurities are likely to surface again at a later time. When this pattern occurs repeatedly, feelings of insecurity and incompetence are likely to emerge. Loss of confidence and self-esteem may quickly follow, resulting in a self-fulfilling prophecy of incompetence and inefficiency. When such individuals become depressed, they experience pervasive feelings of worthlessness and self-deprecation. It may be difficult to shift such depressive thoughts as there may not have been a more adaptive and less critical period in their lives to which reference may be made. People with features of this personality style, when depressed, may become excessively reliant on others to make decisions and to help support them in their day-to-day activities.

Help-seeking may occur at the instigation of a partner or close friend who may become concerned or exhausted at the level of reliance on them. Alternatively, individuals with these personality attributes may realise that they are becoming increasingly dependent on others and that they have lost confidence in their ability to perform simple tasks. In therapy, such individuals pose challenges to recovery in that they may not be familiar with any period in their life when they were not critical of themselves. (Thus, when they present and are asked how long they have been depressed, they often refer 'from birth' and 'forever'). Thus, there may be limited opportunities to utilise previous positive experiences of self-mastery or self-confidence to overcome their present difficulties.

Under stress the Self-critical Personality Style is characterised by:
• Feelings of worthlessness and self-deprecating thoughts.
• Low sense of self-mastery and self-confidence.
• Reliance on others to make decisions and take control.
• Limited opportunities to draw on past positive experiences to overcome present difficulties.

The psychotransmitter model

Our model for psychotransmitter activity suggests that for this personality style, there are significant problems in ion channel activity (e.g. biases towards self-blame and self-criticism) resulting in modification to the types of substances entering the neuron. Within the 'neuron', intracellular mediators (defence mechanisms and coping styles) augment the type and level of stimulation initiated by ion channel activity. Second messengers bear the legacy of these maladaptive processes and switch off self-esteem resulting in depression (Figs 23.1–23.4).

This model relies on the interplay of:
• Modification of substances entering the neuron by faulty ion channels.

Fig. 23.1 Selective attributIONal channels.

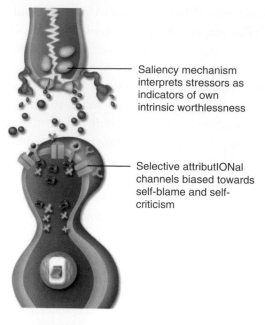

Saliency mechanism interprets stressors as indicators of own intrinsic worthlessness

Selective attributIONal channels biased towards self-blame and self-criticism

Fig. 23.2 Augmentation of faulty ion channel activity.

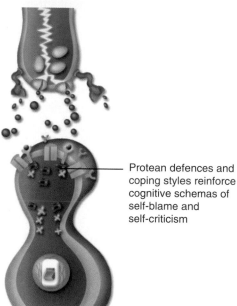

Protean defences and coping styles reinforce cognitive schemas of self-blame and self-criticism

- Intracellular proteins and enzymes which augment faulty ion channel activity.
- Second messengers which bear the legacy of maladaptive intracellular processes.
- Self-esteem gets switched off.

Fig. 23.3 Production
of complex second
messengers.

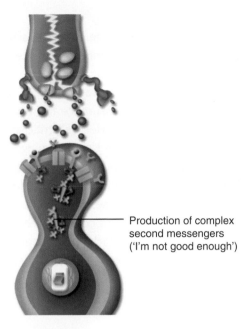

Production of complex
second messengers
('I'm not good enough')

Fig. 23.4 Second
messengers
switch off
self-esteem.

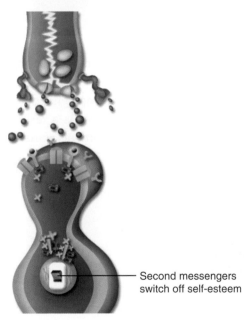

Second messengers
switch off self-esteem

Re-training ion channels (changing faulty attributional and perceptual biases) to respond to other types of ('positive') stimulation from psychotransmitter–receptor complexes is an important aspect of treatment. In addition, it is necessary to prevent the influence of some types of intracellular processes (adverse cognitive schemas) from dominating the production of other second messengers which ultimately switch off self-esteem.

Case vignette – Vanessa

Vanessa was a 37-year-old teacher at a senior school who was well-respected and liked by the other members of the teaching fraternity. She enjoyed her work but found it increasingly difficult to develop new lesson plans as she believed that her innovations were never good enough. Vanessa would constantly seek reassurance from her colleagues for her curriculum development activities. Her self-criticism which sometimes extended to discussing her perceived shortcomings with her colleagues had resulted in several occasions during which she was passed over for promotion in favour of more junior but less self-effacing colleagues who would openly advertise their successes. As the years passed without any advancement in her career, Vanessa's constant self-criticism, especially at her perceived incompetencies and lack of career advancement, wore her down to a state of near exhaustion and she lapsed into an episode of depression. A developmental history identified an uninvolved mother, a critical father and a grandfather who had sexually abused her.

Case summary

Vanessa's depressive episode is the culmination of a series of events which have been shaped by developmental factors and long-standing personality characteristics. Her constant self-criticism has created an impression among her superiors of someone who is incompetent and incapable of holding a more senior position within the school. As a result, she has been overlooked for promotion and her achievements remain unacknowledged by all except those who know her well. Furthermore, her current depressive episode may not only increase her level of self-criticism but also reinforce her perceived incompetence and worthlessness.

Dysfunctional thoughts and attitudes

- I am not as good as others.
- I need others to tell me that my work is all right.
- I cannot cope with responsibility as well as other people.
- Others' reassurance gives me the confidence I lack.

Summary of Vanessa's problem areas

- Low self-esteem and self-confidence.
- Excessive reassurance-seeking among her peers.

- Diminished opportunities because of self-criticism.
- Projection of a negative self-image to others.
- Lack of acknowledgment of strengths and achievements.

Principles of psychological intervention

Medium- to long-term intervention of around 12–20 sessions over a 6-month period with a strong task- and achievement-oriented focus is likely to be helpful. In some cases, therapy may need to be extended over a much longer period. The immediate aims of therapy would be to increase self-esteem and self-confidence, especially in familiar tasks. Specific strategies may involve challenging self-defeating and critical thoughts while engaging in activities with clearly defined outcomes. Discouraging reassurance-seeking behaviours would also form an important component of therapy.

As a personality characteristic, pervasive self-criticism is likely to be embedded in everyday thoughts and behaviours. In long-term therapy it may be necessary to examine how this personality characteristic has shaped previous unfortunate lifestyle choices so that more positive changes may be effected in the future. To this end, it may be useful to embark on setting short- and long-term goals which will gradually change the type and level of life experiences to those that are more fulfilling and less self-defeating. Therapy may also involve family members or close friends who will need to be instructed on providing only minimal reassurance when required.

A structure for psychological intervention
- Medium- to long-term therapy.
- Focus on tasks and clearly defined outcomes.
- Intervention strategies such as challenging self-defeating and critical thoughts.
- Discouraging reassurance-seeking behaviours.
- Goal setting may be helpful in the long-term.
- Involvement of family members and close friends may be helpful.

What sort of therapist?

Support and encouragement, though crucial to establishing rapport, need to be administered without fostering dependency. Individuals with personality features of self-criticism would possibly relate well to a therapist who is open and honest in communication style and likely to work with very clear goals for therapy. Active challenging of dysfunctional attitudes and thoughts by the therapist throughout the therapy process will be necessary to change those entrenched negative beliefs.

Getting started

Depressed individuals with features of a self-critical personality style are likely to seek treatment following a single major life event which has threatened their emotional stability. They may not always be aware of how their long-standing personality characteristics may have contributed to their current state of distress. In setting the aims of therapy, it would be necessary to demonstrate how current thinking and behavioural styles can shape future life experiences. A narrative approach may be especially useful in understanding the problem areas and establishing a framework for therapy. This approach can also be used to identify periods in their life when they overcame specific life stressors using a number of coping skills.

A framework for therapy

A narrative approach requires the therapist to listen to how problems are described as 'stories'. The therapist helps the patient consider how the stories may restrict them from overcoming their present difficulties. The therapist may then contrast these with other 'stories' of previous life crises they handled well and the skills they used in overcoming their difficulties.

For example, the therapist may ask 'What if this happened?' or 'Could it be that this event resulted from X rather than Y?' while posing alternative outcomes to previous life events.

The patient could also be encouraged to document their thoughts about specific life events and the meanings they extracted from those experiences.

The information derived from the first therapy session could be used to shape the treatment plan for future sessions by focusing on specific types of self-criticisms and behavioural and cognitive strategies to actively challenge their veracity. It would also be useful to indicate how present difficulties share similarities with previous problems, especially where excessive self-criticism played a significant role.

Establishing the areas for intervention

At the outset, it would be necessary to forewarn of the possibility of disappointments or setbacks during the course of therapy. Excessive self-criticism in the event of any setbacks can result in the premature discontinuation of therapy. Once a therapy contract is established, however, it is important to adhere to the treatment plan despite possible distractions along the way.

Problem area	Psychological intervention
• Low self-esteem and self-confidence	• Cognitive challenges of dysfunctional thoughts, and behavioural 'experiments'
• Excessive reassurance-seeking among peers	• Response prevention and distraction strategies
• Diminished opportunities because of self-criticism	• Active pursuit of opportunities and new experiences
• Projection of a negative self-image to others	• Self-praise or discussion of achievements to others
• Lack of acknowledgment of strengths and achievements	• Self-reward for task completion

Intervention strategies

1. Cognitive challenges and behavioural 'experiments' to test the veracity of dysfunctional thoughts are useful strategies that should be used throughout the course of therapy. Cognitive challenges would mainly take the form of identifying and challenging negative self-statements and criticisms.

Identifying and challenging negative self-statements

Identify the negative self-statement, then narrow it down to a specific instance or example before challenging it:

General self-statement	Specific self-statement	Challenging self-statement
'I am worthless'	'I can't cook well and that makes me feel worthless'	'Being a poor cook doesn't mean I'm worthless. I can do other things well'

Behavioural 'experiments' can also be used to challenge negative self-statements and criticisms by actively encouraging the acknowledgment of expertise in an area. For example, a hierarchy of tasks could be developed so that achievements can be operationalised and measured over a specified time period. At the completion of each activity it would be useful to ask how the task has changed any negative self-perceptions.

2. Response prevention and distraction strategies may be used to actively discourage reassurance-seeking behaviours. Identify situations where reassurance-seeking would be likely, then consider alternate activities which could be engaged in until the anxieties have dissipated. Response prevention strategies could involve not using the telephone for a few hours or not visiting a friend until the urge to seek reassurance has passed. Distraction strategies could involve engaging in any activity such as a hobby or sporting activity that distracts from those anxieties.

3. It may be useful to encourage a new and interesting activity on a weekly basis in order to explore potential areas of expertise that may not have otherwise been considered. For example, interests and hobbies of child-hood or early adulthood could be re-visited. Alternatively, magazines or newspapers could be scoured for interesting new challenges.

4. While it may seem somewhat contrived, it may be necessary to encourage active self-promotion among colleagues and friends. This can be role-played, firstly during the course of therapy before in vivo practice. Positive self-statements or statements of achievement could be actively worked into the course of conversation without appearing staged or artificial. These may take the form of 'I am good at … ' or 'I am so pleased that I have done … '.

5. Self-reward strategies involve making obvious any tasks that, in their completion, serve to dispute negative self-statement and self-perceptions. Graphs or star-charts may be used to mark the successful completion or execution of such activities. Self-reward in the form of small treats, engagement in pleasurable activities or pastimes can also be used to mark success.

Building resilience

Developing expertise and acknowledging success in one or more activities, however trivial, can help build self-confidence. Over time, these achievements can be strung together to challenge global and negative cognitive schemas. Another useful strategy is to learn to 'isolate' or 'quarantine' stressors so that they do not impinge on self-esteem. This requires deconstructing each stressor into its component parts and dealing with each part separately using problem-solving strategies.

Barriers to effective intervention

One of the potential difficulties in treating people with features of a self-critical personality style may be the lack of insight about the influence of such characteristics on the development of depression. Therapy may need to proceed at a slower pace and be extended over a longer period in order to effect substantial and persistent change.

The role of medication

We are not persuaded that antidepressant medication has a primary role for individuals who are depressed as a consequence of this personality style, although the selective serotonin reuptake inhibitors (SSRIs) may ease some depressive features and allow the individual to feel less stressed and more 'swimming than sinking' if anxiety is significant. We view psychosocial intervention as likely to be of far greater use than a medication-based approach.

24

Natural and alternative treatments for non-melancholic depression

It has been estimated that up to 50% of Australians who suffer from a depressive disorder may seek self-help or non-medical complementary treatments for their condition. The popularity of natural and alternative treatment lies in their easy availability and low cost, positive associations with optimal health, and social acceptability. Other reasons for their popularity may relate to feelings of self-efficacy and self-direction in matters of personal health and well-being.

Natural and alternative treatments are those practices that are not within the range of mainstream acceptable treatments. Research has indicated that these practices may have some efficacy for some presentations of non-melancholic depression, but are unlikely to be of primary benefit to those who suffer from melancholic or psychotic depression or bipolar disorder.

The range of natural and alternate treatments

There are many types of natural and alternate treatments for depressive disorders, some of which are only just beginning to gain credibility among professionals and the mainstream medical establishment. With the exception of a handful of treatments, the clinical efficacy of the vast majority of these treatments has not yet been empirically determined in randomised controlled trials (RCTs). Furthermore, it is only possible to speculate on how personality features in non-melancholic depression may affect the use of natural and alternative treatments, treatment compliance, and clinical efficacy.

Some of the more commonly used natural and alternative treatments have been grouped into three categories described as follows:

1. *Therapies which advocate lifestyle and behaviour change*: These include the adoption of specific methods for relaxation and distraction from distress, as well as modifications to the immediate environment and changes in lifestyle.

2. *Non-prescription medicines*: Including over-the-counter preparations and herbs, foodstuffs, and vitamins.
3. *Dietary changes*: Usually involving the cessation or reduction of specific foods in the diet.

Lifestyle and behaviour change

Acupressure

This technique uses many of the acupoints as acupuncture with deep finger pressure instead of needles. The technique appears to be effective for stress-related conditions including some types of depressive disorders. Acupressure may be self-administered and used in conjunction with deep breathing, which helps to release tension and improve the flow of energy throughout the body.

Acupuncture

This traditional Chinese treatment involves the insertion of fine needles into specific points in the body in order to correct energy imbalances. The needles may be manipulated by hand or stimulated electrically (electro-acupuncture), the latter considered to be the more effective procedure. A series of studies (Han & Terenius, 1982) investigating the putative mechanism of action for acupuncture has found that endorphin levels can be increased through needling, and that it has some antidepressant benefit to some individuals as a consequence of that factor. Controlled trials conducted in China have argued that electro-acupuncture is as effective as tricyclic antidepressants (Han, 1986; Luo et al., 1998) but the treatment requires further clinical investigation.

Air ionisation

It is hypothesised that negative air ions, which decrease in autumn and winter, are related to a concomitant decrease in brain serotonin levels. Electrical devices have been developed which can increase the concentration of negative air ions as a treatment for winter depression. Two studies (Terman & Terman, 1995; Terman et al., 1998) have demonstrated the effectiveness of high density air ionisation in the treatment of winter depression but not for other types of depression.

Alcohol for relaxation

While recent surveys have demonstrated that moderate drinkers have lower levels of depressive symptoms than non-drinkers, the reasons for these findings are unknown (Lipton, 1994; Rodgers et al., 2000). It is recognised that alcohol has mood-enhancing effects but the quantity consumed and the circumstances surrounding consumption can enhance its effects. At present, there is insufficient evidence to draw any firm conclusion about the benefits of alcohol in alleviating depression.

Aromatherapy

Heated plant oils, such as bergamot, geranium, chamomile, lavender and rosemary, are allowed to diffuse in a room or used as components of massage oils and are said to help alleviate depressive moods. These oils are thought to have specific psychopharmacological properties once absorbed through the skin. Although there is no evidence to support its use in the treatment of depression, aromatherapy is often used in conjunction with massage, the combined efficacy of which is declared by some patients.

Art therapy

Art therapy is thought to help people express feelings that they would otherwise experience difficulty in doing. Paintings, drawings, and other forms of creative expression are thought to reflect the patient's personality, conflicts, concerns, and interests. It is thought that this form of therapy may help to resolve conflicts, improve self-esteem, and facilitate personal development and emotional growth. Its efficacy in achieving these aims remains to be determined however.

Bibliotherapy

In this form of treatment, patients are given standardised treatments in books and told to work through them on their own with intermittent reviews with a mental health professional. Bibliotherapy tends to be effective when applied to cognitive-behavioural therapy, possibly because this form of therapy lends itself more easily to a structured approach. Although evidence supports its effectiveness, it requires a good reading level in order to derive the most benefits. Also, it may not be useful for those whose depressive mood has resulted in severe problems in attention and concentration.

Colour therapy

Broad expanses of colour in the environment are thought to influence mood states. Changing the colours in one's environment by re-painting or re-decorating the home or office, though unproven, is held to be of some benefit by some individuals when depressed (and presumably more for 'normal' rather than for clinical depression).

Dance and movement

This form of therapy encourages patients to express themselves through dance and movement. The rationale is that expressing feelings through movement can have a positive effect on mood. If conducted in a group, dance therapy has the additional element of encouraging social interaction, which could be helpful to depressed patients. No specific mechanism for the putative beneficial effects of dance therapy has been proposed; however, the physical exercise involved in this form of therapy may, in itself, be beneficial to some individuals.

Enjoyable activities

The reason for engaging in pleasant activities is to improve mood and distract from negative or distressing thoughts. People who are suffering from a depressive illness tend to engage in fewer pleasant activities, thus reducing opportunities for relief from their distress. This strategy is often used in conjunction with cognitive-behaviour therapy or interpersonal skills training but there is little evidence for its effectiveness when used alone.

Exercise

While regular (aerobic) exercise improves strength, flexibility, and stamina, it also helps to relieve some muscle tension due to anxiety and stress. Exercise can interrupt ruminative thoughts, provide a distraction from unwanted negative thoughts, and increase social interaction if conducted in a group environment. Strenuous exercise, such as aerobic exercise, promotes the release of endorphins, the body's natural opiates. As fitness levels are known to be reduced in depressed individuals, it has been argued that increased aerobic fitness may directly lift mood. Several studies have attested to the benefits of exercise in alleviating depressive symptoms (Babyak et al., 2000; Singh et al., 2001).

Laughter therapy

Research has shown that laughter can boost the functioning of the immune system, reduce anxiety, and distract from chronic pain or other debilitating physical illnesses. One theory is that laughter causes the brain to produce endorphins, which helps to ease pain and lift mood. However, there are no studies on the effects of laughter therapy on alleviating depressive disorder.

LeShan distance healing

This technique developed by LeShan, a psychologist, is based on the premise that healing occurs naturally when the healer is in an altered state of consciousness and meditates on the depressed individual. Only one RCT has examined LeShan distance healing as an adjunct to psychiatric treatment for major depression and found no significant effect (Greyson, 1996).

Light therapy

The reduced availability of sunlight in winter is hypothesised to cause a phase delay in circadian rhythms which, in susceptible people, can lead to depression. Treatment involves exposure to a bank of bright lights for about an hour a day, preferably in the morning, a procedure which is thought to correct the phase delay. This treatment is effective for seasonal depression or winter depression with patterns of response dependent on the brightness level of the lights (Lee & Chan, 1999). This treatment has also been shown to be effective for non-seasonal depression although the evidence is limited (Kripke, 1998).

Massage

Massage involves the therapeutic manipulation of soft tissue and is thought to affect depression by shifting electroencephalogram activity from a right frontal pattern (associated with dysthymic affect) to a left frontal or symmetrical pattern (associated with euthymic affect). Furthermore, massage increases vagal activity and stimulates facial expressions and vocalisations, which helps lessen depressive affect. Limited evidence suggests that massage is beneficial in alleviating some symptoms of depression in the short term.

Meditation and yoga

Meditation and many forms of yoga involve the process of focusing one's attention on a word, a thought, an image, an idea or some other concept which induces a state of relaxation. While meditation techniques tend to be used in the treatment of stress and anxiety conditions, their ability to reduce arousal levels makes them useful for some types of depressive disorders. Meditation and yoga as treatments for depression have yet to be fully evaluated, although limited investigations on yogic breathing look promising.

Music

Due to its ability to arouse strong emotions, music has been tried as a therapy for depression. Studies have demonstrated that, when accompanied by other interventions, it can help to relieve pain through distraction, lower blood pressure, and reduce anxiety and depression. Music is hypothesised to affect frontal and limbic system functioning, although the mechanism by which this occurs is unknown. The type of music chosen for each session of music therapy depends on the age, personality and preference of the patient. When used in combination with other interventions such as cognitive-behaviour therapy or antidepressants, music seems to have some therapeutic effect. However, as yet no evidence exists that listening to music on its own helps to relieve depression.

Pets

Pets can provide companionship and a sense of responsibility for people suffering from a depressive illness. There is also anecdotal evidence to suggest that pet ownership is beneficial to physical and mental well-being. Pets can reduce a sense of isolation and provide companionship. Limited research has demonstrated that stroking a dog or a cat can lower blood pressure, heart rate, and respiratory rate, and people with coronary heart disease who own pets have better survival rates than those who do not, although the pattern is not always consistent. However, to date there have been no methodologically sound studies examining the long-term therapeutic benefits of pet ownership on the course and outcome of a depressive episode.

Prayer

This traditional form of healing has been used to gain relief from many illnesses and life-style problems including depression. Some studies (e.g. Koenig et al., 1998) have demonstrated that those who attended religious services once a week were less likely to become depressed. One study of hospitalised medical patients with depression (Koenig, 1999) indicated that those with higher scores on an index of religiosity were more likely to recover faster from their depression than those who scored low on that questionnaire. However, the efficacy of prayer is impossible to determine as it is dependent upon several non-measurable variables such as level of social support, which could contribute to its potential success.

Relaxation therapy

These include a number of techniques, such as progressive muscle relation, to teach voluntarily muscle relaxation. Although initially developed as a method to control stress and anxiety by decreasing physical and mental tension, relaxation techniques are used in the treatment of depression especially where there is significant co-morbidity. It is usually used in conjunction with other types of therapy such as cognitive-behaviour therapy and antidepressant medication. There is some evidence to indicate that it is effective in the treatment of depressive disorders but more research is needed in larger studies with long-term follow-up.

Improving sleep

While disturbed sleep can be one of the symptoms of a depressive disorder, sleep problems may also exacerbate a depressive episode. The most common types of sleep problems include difficulty in going to sleep, staying asleep and early morning awakening. There are a number of techniques that can be used to improve the quality of sleep including establishing a bedtime ritual, drinking a warm glass of milk, engaging in relaxing activities before bedtime, dimming the lights a few hours before going to sleep, and using relaxation or meditation exercises to help wind down.

Non-prescription medicines

Fish oils

Omega 3 fatty acids (O3FAs) such as those found in fish are thought to be important in nervous system functioning. Low concentrations of one of the fatty acids found in oily fish has been associated with low concentrations of a serotonin metabolite found in cerebrospinal fluid which, in turn, has been associated with depression and suicide. There are now published trials suggesting benefit from O3FAs for bipolar disorder (Stoll et al., 1999) and as augmenting antidepressant drugs in treatment resistant depression (Nemets et al., 2002; Peet, 2003).

Ginseng

Extracts from the root of this plant are used in several different types of preparations including an infusion to improve energy levels and vigour. Ginseng is thought to stimulate adrenal gland activity and thus increase overall energy levels. It is also thought to help the body cope with stress but its effect as an antidepressant has yet to be demonstrated.

Ginkgo

This product is derived from the leaves of a tree and is available in tablet form. It has been used for treating impaired cerebral circulation, the symptoms of which are similar to those of depressive disorders. A typical dose is 40 mg three times per day or 80 mg twice per day. Except for one trial on the prevention of seasonal affective disorder (Linjaerde et al., 1999), in which ginkgo was found to be ineffective, there have not been any other clinical trials on depressed individuals.

Glutamine

This amino acid is the precursor of the neurotransmitter glutamate, the synthesis of which appears to be affected in depression. Glutamate is thought to increase energy levels and improve mood but there has not been any clear clinical evidence to support its use.

Homoeopathy

Physical and psychological symptoms are thought to reflect the way in which the body attempts to 'heal' itself. Rather than aiming to eliminate symptoms, this type of treatment involves the administration of dilute concentrations of substances which produce the same symptoms in an attempt to mobilise the body's own healing power. There is no clear clinical evidence to demonstrate its effectiveness in the treatment of depression.

Kava kava

This herb, which is a member of the pepper family, is used to treat depressive disorders when anxiety plays a significant role in presentation. The herb has been used by the South Pacific polynesians in traditional ceremonies and as a muscle relaxant, sedative, and anxiolytic for over 3000 years. The dose of kava is usually around 100 mg for anxiety and 200 mg for sleep problems. Its antidepressant effects have not been evaluated as rigorously as those for St John's wort.

Lemon balm

Lemon balm tea has traditionally been used for its antidepressant effects which lift mood and counter feelings of lethargy and apathy but, so far, these claims have not been evaluated. The recommended dose is three to four cups of tea per day or half to one teaspoon of tincture up to three times per day.

Natural progesterone

Natural progesterone is available as a cream or as a suppository and differs from synthetic progestogens. It is thought to influence serotonergic function in the brain and has been postulated as a treatment for depressive disorders related to hormonal imbalance, such as postnatal, premenstrual, perimenstrual, perimenopausal, and postmenopausal depression. The few trials that have been conducted on women diagnosed with premenstrual syndrome have not found any evidence to suggest that it improves mood.

Painkillers

Many people report taking painkillers to alleviate their mood when depressed. In high doses, codeine (a narcotic) can have some mood-enhancing effects and there is speculation that aspirin may also have some mood-modulating effects. However, the treatment efficacy of painkillers is yet to be evaluated.

Phenylalanine

This essential amino acid is a precursor of catecholamine neurotransmitters. There have only been a small number of studies examining the efficacy of this substance on treating depressive disorders and in one study it was found to work as well as imipramine (Beckmann et al., 1979).

Selenium

Subclinical deficiencies of this essential trace element are thought to affect mood. Although there is some evidence to suggest that selenium supplements can improve mood in normal subjects (Benton & Cook, 1991), there is no evidence to support selenium supplementation in the treatment of depressive disorders.

S-adenosylmethionine

This amino acid derivative occurs naturally in all cells and is thought to play a role in many biological processes including neurotransmitter metabolism and receptor functioning. Its use is contraindicated, unless otherwise stated, for people suffering from a bipolar depressive disorder and using prescription antidepressants. Studies are encouraging and demonstrate that more depressed patients respond to S-adenosylmethionine (SAMe) than to placebos although studies comparing it to tricyclics have not found any differences. SAMe seldom has side-effects, which make it more tolerable than some of the older antidepressants. However, further research is required to test its efficacy against the newer antidepressants.

St John's wort

Hypericum perforatum or St John's wort, a plant extract, has gained in popularity in the treatment of depressive disorders because of its relatively benign side effects and low drug–drug interactions. The herb is widely used in Europe and is slowly gaining acceptance in North America and Australia despite some reports that it is no more effective than placebo. However, such negative reports may be due to problems in its inappropriate use in some subtypes of depressive disorders. Its efficacy is thought to be related to the inhibition of the synaptic reuptake of serotonin, norepinephrine, and dopamine. A therapeutic dose is around 300 mg taken three times per day at mealtimes. It may take anywhere between 3 and 6 weeks to derive the anti-depressant effects of the herb. St John's wort is reported to have fewer side-effects than conventional prescription antidepressants. However, it can interact with other medications including selective serotonin reuptake inhibitors (SSRIs) and other drugs. While seemingly as effective as many of the new antidepressants (as reviewed in Chapter 1) for some depressive disorders, such a conclusion is likely to be confounded by the current designs and practices of RCTs.

Tyrosine

Tyrosine, an amino acid produced from phenylalanine, is a precursor of catecholamine neurotransmitters. One study (Gelenberg et al., 1990) comparing tyrosine with imipramine and placebo found no evidence for its use as an antidepressant.

Valerian

This herb, which acts as a mild tranquiliser, has a long history of use in the treatment of insomnia and stress-related symptoms. It is thought to act on the neurotransmitter systems for serotonin and gamma aminobutyric acid, which help regulate mood, sleep and level of relaxation. The recommended dose for depressive symptoms is between 300 and 500 mg taken around an hour before bedtime.

Vervain

This flowering plant has been traditionally used to treat depression but its effectiveness remains to be examined.

Vitamins

It is hypothesised that folate and vitamins B6 and B12 may facilitate the synthesis of the chemical precursors of serotonin, dopamine, and norepinephrine. Vitamin D levels, which decrease during the winter months, are thought to play a role in the development of winter depression. There is tentative evidence to suggest that folate may be effective, either as a primary treatment or as an augmentor, in some types of depressive disorders. Other vitamins (e.g., the antioxidants, vitamin D, and vitamin E) are also thought to improve mood but there is insufficient evidence to demonstrate a clear therapeutic role in depression treatment.

Dietary changes

Alcohol avoidance or reduction

Evidence has demonstrated that heavy drinkers and those with alcohol dependence disorders have an increased risk of suffering from a depressive disorder. This may be attributable to the direct effects of alcohol or it may result from secondary problems, such as financial, occupational, relationship and health problems, associated with alcohol misuse. However, there is no evidence to suggest that alcohol avoidance or reduction is effective for treating depression in people who do not have problems with alcohol misuse or dependence.

Caffeine avoidance or reduction

Some individuals are thought to be sensitive to the effects of caffeine, found in coffee and cola drinks, which, in turn, leads to depression. There is evidence to suggest that caffeine increases anxiety in individuals who experience panic attacks. Its reported effect on precipitating depressive disorders may be largely due to its frequent co-occurrence with anxiety.

Chocolate

The possible antidepressant effects of chocolate have recently received much media interest. Speculation abounds on the mode of antidepressant action including its high carbohydrate content, which is thought to contribute to increased serotonin production. The many psychoactive substances such as caffeine, phenylethylamine, and theobromide found in chocolate are also thought to contribute to alleviating depressed mood. In addition, chocolate has many pleasant sensory characteristics, which are thought to stimulate the release of endorphins.

Sugar avoidance or reduction

Some people are thought to be sensitive to the highs ('sugar highs') and lows (low blood sugar levels) associated with sucrose which is thought to lead to depression. Such individuals report feeling fatigued and moody, suffer from headaches, sleep more than usual, and feel tense and irritable. Reducing the intake of sucrose has been found to be beneficial for some depressed individuals but further research in this area is needed, and the hypothesis has yet to be substantiated.

Summary

Lack of empirical evidence makes it difficult to evaluate the relative efficacy of most natural and alternative treatments. The most popular treatments with the best evidence for effectiveness are St John's wort, physical exercise, self-help books, and light therapy for winter depression. However, while there are some well-designed outcome studies on complementary and self-help treatment, in general many of the studies are poorly designed with small sample sizes, short periods of follow-up, non-random selection of subjects, and poor outcome measures.

Limited evidence suggests that these treatments, usually provided in combination, would be effective for some expressions of non-melancholic depression but are unlikely to be of primary benefit in melancholic and psychotic depression. Some of these treatments, especially the non-prescription medicines, require a degree of understanding or judgement but allow sufferers to take more control over their treatment. Other treatments, such as those involving alternate healers (acupuncturists, masseurs, etc), may not require such knowledge about the procedure itself but may require patients to relinquish control to another person (the alternate healer) in order to effect a cure.

While many natural and alternative treatments may be of assistance to most expressions of non-melancholic depression, specific types of such treatments may have differing efficacy across varying personality styles. For example, changing lifestyle to alleviate distress would probably appeal to those with heightened levels of arousal (such as those with the personality features of anxious worrying and irritability). Those with high levels of self-criticism, perfectionism, and interpersonal sensitivity may also benefit from some modifications in lifestyle. People with high levels of perfectionism and self-criticism may be more likely to use non-prescription medications to overcome depression. However, those with features of anxious worrying may also prefer to find relief in non-prescription medications and herbal remedies. Dietary changes may appeal to those with the personality features of irritability and perfectionism, while those with self-focused features may be less likely to resort to natural and alternative treatments.

Appendix 1: The DMI-18 and the DMI-10

The 18-item Depression in the Medically Ill (DMI-18) and the briefer DMI-10 (Parker et al., 2001a, b), were originally developed as short-screening measures. Items are independent of medical illness features, as many (e.g. sleep disturbance, appetite disturbance, and weight change) overlap with physiological symptoms of depression. Thus, only 'cognitive-based' items reflecting the mood state of depression are included while somatic symptoms are excluded.

Items are scored on a 4-point scale, where a score of 0 indicates the statement is 'not true'; 1, 'slightly true'; 2, 'moderately true'; and 3, 'very true'. Individual item scores are summed to derive a total depression score. For the extended version, the DMI-18, a cut-off of 20 or more is indicative of probable or definite depression while, for the briefer DMI-10, a score of 9 or more is suggestive of probable or definite depression.

The measure has also been tested on a large sample of over 600 patients attending general practitioners, where its utility as a screening measure of state depression has been established (Parker et al., 2001c). Criterion-related validity was reflected in the high sensitivity (94–100% for the DMI-10 and 92–95% for the DMI-18) and specificity estimates (66–70% for the DMI-10 and 68–72% for the DMI-18) of the measure against two criteria: the clinical judgement of a psychiatrist, and the computer-generated Diagnostic and Statistical Manual of Mental Disorder (DSM-IV) diagnosis from the Composite International Diagnostic Interview (CIDI) (World Health Organization, 1997; Parker et al., 2001b).

Internal consistency measured by Cronbach's alpha is high for both the DMI-10 (0.89) and DMI-18 (0.93) in medical inpatients (Parker et al., 2001b). Cronbach's alpha for the DMI-10 was 0.92 (Parker et al., 2001b) in a general practice setting. Both scales also have high-convergent validity with two other depression scales, namely the BDI-PC (Beck Depression Inventory for Primary Care) and the HADS (the Hospital Anxiety and Depression Scale). The DMI-10 returned Spearman correlations of 0.80

with the BDI-PC and 0.70 with the HADS while the DMI-18 returned correlations of 0.78 with the BDI-PC and 0.72 with the HADS (Parker et al., 2001b).

The final self-report measure takes little time to complete and is acceptable to patients in general hospitals, those attending their general practitioner and psychiatric outpatients. A recent study has demonstrated that scores on the DMI-10, which are also independent of gender, can be used to reliably assign depression caseness in outpatients attending psychiatric services (Parker & Gladstone, 2004). Scores exceeding cut-off values, in combination with usual duration and impairment criteria, allow a useful estimate of the likelihood of clinical depression. The instruments are available for general use through the Black Dog Institute web site (www.blackdoginstitute.org.au).

Appendix 2: The CORE system of measuring psychomotor disturbance

The CORE was initially developed as a measure of the domains of psychomotor disturbance specific to melancholic and psychotic depressive disorders. A full description of its developmental is provided in Parker and Hadzi-Pavlovic (1996). The final measure comprises 18 signs (observable features) which are rated by the clinician or a trained observer at the end of a clinical interview. Each sign is rated on a 4-point scale (0–3), where a rating of 0 conveys a general concept of normality or the subject's usual behaviour. By contrast, a rating of 2 or 3 always implies definite pathological behaviour. A score of 3 also indicates severe disturbance on that behavioural domain. Sub-sets of items produce scores on each of three dimensions found to underlie psychomotor change: 'non-interactiveness', 'retardation', and 'agitation'.

Principal components analysis of the 18 items of the CORE suggested a trunk and branch analogy for construing psychomotor disturbance and for deriving subscales. The six truncal items contribute to a non-interactiveness scale which is thought to reflect disturbances in neurocognitive processing or the psychic component of psychomotor disturbance, which, when severe, can generate a diagnosis of pseudo-dementia in depressed patients. The remaining CORE items on the left- and right-hand 'branches' define the motor aspects of psychomotor disturbance, with some specificity to either agitation or to retardation. The CORE measure may be used in three principal ways:

(i)   as a total CORE score, and thus as a dimensional measure of psychomotor disturbance;
(ii) as three dimensional sub-scale scores (i.e. non-interactiveness, agitation, and retardation);
(iii) to generate categories of likely melancholic and non-melancholic depression (i.e. using a total CORE score of 8 or more).

Inter-rater reliability for the presence or absence of individual items and item severity scores following training were found to be high (kappa values of up to 0.61 and intraclass correlations of up to 0.87) in samples of depressed patients in Australia and the USA. Significant dose–response relationships were found between dexamethasone non-suppression and CORE scores. These findings are consistent with an extensive literature indicating that psychomotor disturbance is the most replicable clinical correlate of dexamethasone non-suppression. In another series of studies, melancholic and non-melancholic depressives were differentiated strongly by CORE scores. Melancholic depressives so identified demonstrated significant and specific neuropsychological deficits evident from extensive psychometric testing, as well as demonstrating higher rates of lesions in magnetic resonance imaging. Further information about the psychometric properties of the measure is reported in Parker and Hadzi-Pavlovic (1996). The CORE measure and rating instructions are also available through the Black Dog Institute web site (www.blackdoginstitute.org.au).

Appendix 3: The temperament and personality measure

The 109-item temperament and personality (T&P) measure assesses both personality characteristics (8 subscales) and disordered functioning (2 subscales). Items for assessing T&P were selected from a larger item pool and, were included only if their factor loadings were high and after consideration of their clinical usefulness as 'markers' of that particular construct.

Each item of the T&P measure is rated on a 4-point scale where 'not true at all' is assigned a rating of 1; 'slightly true', 2; 'moderately true', 3; and 'very true', 4. To obtain judgements about trait characteristics, subjects are asked to tick the rating option 'that best describes the way you usually or generally feel or behave' (over the years and not just recently). Subscale scores for each of the 8 T&P dimensions are derived by summing the relevant items for that subscale and compared against a set of norms. The 8 subscales are as follows:

(i)   Anxious worrying (8 items)
(ii)   Perfectionism (8 items)
(iii)   Personal reserve (8 items)
(iv)   Irritability (8 items)
(v)   Social avoidance (7 items)
(vi)   Sensitivity to rejection (7 items)
(vii)   Self-criticism (8 items)
(viii) Self-focused (7 items).

Psychometric properties of the measure have been established in a number of studies on samples including general practice attenders, psychiatric outpatients suffering from a depressive disorder, and a web-based community survey of 'ever depressed' participants. Except for the self-focused subscale, all other subscales correlate highly with clinician ratings of personality style (correlations range from 0.35 to 0.54). Test–retest reliabilities at 3 weeks for the subscales were high with intraclass correlations ranging from 0.65 (self-focused) to 0.93 (social avoidance).

The T&P measure is available for general use through the Black Dog Institute web site (www.blackdoginstitute.org.au).

References

Akiskal, H. S., & McKinney Jr., W. T. (1975). Overview of recent research in depression. Integration of ten conceptual models into a comprehensive clinical frame. *Archives of General Psychiatry, 32*(3), 285–305.

Altschule, M. D. (1967). The two kinds of depression according to St. Paul. *British Journal of Psychiatry, 113,* 779–780.

American Psychiatric Association. (1980). *Diagnostic and statistical manual of mental disorders (DSM-III)* (3rd ed.). Washington, DC: American Psychiatric Association.

American Psychiatric Association. (1994). *Diagnostic and statistical manual of mental disorders (DSM-IV)* (4th ed.). Washington, DC: American Psychiatric Association.

American Psychiatric Association. (2000). *APA practice guidelines for the treatment of psychiatric disorders, compendium 2000.* Washington, DC: American Psychiatric Association.

Anderson, I. M. (2000). Selective serotonin reuptake inhibitors versus tricyclic antidepressants: a meta-analysis of efficacy and tolerability. *Journal of Affective Disorders, 58*(1), 19–36.

Babyak, M., Blumenthal, J. A., Herman, S., Khatri, P., Doraiswamy, M., Moore, K., et al. (2000). Exercise treatment for major depression: maintenance of therapeutic benefit at 10 months. *Psychosomatic Medicine, 62*(5), 633–638.

Beck, A. T. (1983). Cognitive therapy of depression: new perspectives. In J. Barrett (Ed.), *Treatment of depression: old controversies and new approaches* (pp. 265–290). New York, NY: Raven press.

Beck, A. T., Rush, A. J., Shaw, B. F., & Emery, G. (1979). *Cognitive therapy of depression.* New York, NY: Guilford.

Beckmann, H., Athen, D., Olteanu, M., & Zimmer, R. (1979). DL-phenylalanine versus imipramine: a double-blind study. *Archiv fur Psychiatrie Nervenkrankheiten, 227,* 49–58.

Benton, D., & Cook, R. (1991). The impact of selenium supplementation on mood. *Biological Psychiatry, 29*(11), 1092–1098.

Blashfield, R. K., & Morey, L. C. (1979). The classification of depression through cluster analysis. *Comprehensive Psychiatry, 20,* 516–527.

Boyce, P., & Parker, G. (1989). Development of a scale to measure interpersonal sensitivity. *Australian & New Zealand Journal of Psychiatry, 23*(3), 341–351.

Bryson, B. (2003). *A short history of nearly everything.* Sydney: Doubleday.

Carroll, B. J. (1989). Diagnostic validity and laboratory studies: rules of the game. In J. E. Barrett (Ed.), *The validity of psychiatric diagnosis* (pp. 229–245). New York, NY: Raven Press.

Costa, P. T., & McCrae, R. R. (1990). Personality disorders and the five-factor model of personality. *Journal of Personality Disorders, 4*(4), 362–371.

Costa, P. T., & McRae, R. R. (1992). *Revised NEO personality inventory (NEO PI-R) and NEO five-factor inventory (NEO-FFI) professional manual.* Odessa, FL: Psychological Assessment Resources.

Deveson, A. (2003). *Resilience.* Sydney: Allen & Unwin.

DHHS Depression Guideline Panel. (1993). *Depression in primary care. Volume 2. Treatment of major depression.* Rockville, MD: US Department of Health and Human Services. Public Health Service, Agency or Health Care Policy and Research.

Epstein, D., & White, M. (1992). *Experience, contradiction, narrative and imagination. Selected papers of David Epstein and Michael White.* Adelaide: Dulwich Centre Publications.

Erikson, E. H. (1995). *Childhood and society* (2nd ed.). London: Vintage.

Furman, B., & Ahola, T. (1994). Solution talk: the solution-oriented way of talking about problems. In M. F. Hoyt (Ed.), *Constructive therapies.* New York, NY: The Guilford Press.

Geertz, C. (1975). *The interpretation of cultures.* London: Hutchinson.

Gelenberg, A. J., Wojcik, J. D., Falk, W. E., Baldessarini, R. J., et al. (1990). Tyrosine for depression: A double-blind trial. *Journal of Affective Disorders, 19*(2), 125–132.

Goodwin, G. M., Anderson, I., Angst, J., Baldwin, D., Bhagwagar, Z., Cookson, J., et al. (2003). Evidence-based guidelines for treating bipolar disorder: recommendations from the British Association for Psychopharmacology. *Journal of Psychopharmacology, 17*(2), 149–173.

Greyson, B. (1996). Distance healing of patients with major depression. *Journal of Science Exploration, 10,* 447–465.

Hadjipavlou, G., Mok, H., & Yatham, L. N. (2004). Bipolar II disorder: an overview of recent developments. *Canadian Journal of Psychiatry, 49,* 802–812.

Hamilton, M. (1960). A rating scale for depression. *Journal of Neurology, Neuroscience and Psychiatry, 23,* 56.

Han, J. S. (1986). Electroacupuncture: an alternative to antidepressants for treating affective diseases? *International Journal of Neuroscience, 29*(1–2), 79–92.

Han, J. S., & Terenius, L. (1982). Neurochemical basis for acupuncture analgesia. *Annual Review of Pharmacology and Toxicology, 22,* 193–220.

Himmelhoch, J. M. (2003). On the usefulness of clinical case studies: commentary. *Bipolar Disorders, 5*(1), 69–71.

Holmes, J. (2002). All you need is cognitive behaviour therapy. *British Medical Journal, 324,* 288–294.

Hypericum Depression Trial Study Group. (2002). Effect of Hypericum perforatum (St John's wort) in major depressive disorder: a randomized controlled trial. *Journal of the American Medical Association, 287*(14), 1807–1814.

Ivey, A. (1988). *Intentional interviewing and counselling – facilitating client development* (2nd ed.). California, CA: Brooks/Cole Publishing Company.

Jackson, S. W. (1986). *Melancholia and depression: from hippocratic times to modern times*. New Haven and London: Yale University Press.

Khan, A., Khan, S., & Brown, W. A. (2002). Are placebo controls necessary to test new antidepressants and anxiolytics? *International Journal of Neuropsychopharmacology, 5*(3), 193–197.

Kiloh, L. G., Andrews, G., Neilson, M., & Bianchi, G. N. (1972). The relationship of the syndromes called endogenous and neurotic depression. *British Journal of Psychiatry, 121*(561), 183–196.

Kirk, S. A., & Kutchins, H. (1992). *The selling of DSM: the rhetoric of science in psychiatry*. New York, NY: Aldine de Gruyter.

Kirsch, I., Moore, T. J., Scoboria, A., & Nicholls, S. (2002). The Emperor's new drugs: an analysis of antidepressant medication data, submitted to the US Food and Drug Administration. *Prevention and Treatment, 5*, 1–11.

Klerman, G. L., & Weissman, M. M. (1994). *Interpersonal psychotherapy of depression*. London: Jason Aronson, Inc.

Koenig, H. G. (1999). Religious attitudes and practices of hospitalized medically ill adults. *International Journal of Geriatric Psychiatry, 13*(4), 213–224.

Koenig, H. G., George, L. K., & Peterson, B. L. (1998). Religiosity and remission of depression in medically ill older patients. *American Journal of Psychiatry, 155*(4), 536–542.

Kripke, D. F. (1998). Light treatment for nonseasonal depression: speed, efficacy, and combined treatment. *Journal of Affective Disorders, 49*(2), 109–117.

Kruedelbach, N., McCormick, R. A., Schulz, S., & Grueneich, R. (1993). Impulsivity, coping styles, and triggers for craving in substance abusers with borderline personality disorder. *Journal of Personality Disorders, 7*(3), 214–222.

Lee, T. M. C., & Chan, C. C. H. (1999). Dose–response relationship of phototherapy for seasonal affective disorder: a meta-analysis. *Acta Psychiatrica Scandinavica, 99*(5), 315–323.

Lewis, A. J. (1931). *A clinical and historical survey of depressive states based on the study of 61 cases*. Unpublished Ph.D., University of Adelaide, Adelaide.

Linjaerde, O., Foreland, A. R., & Magnusson, A. (1999). Can winter depression be prevented by *Ginkgo biloba* extract? A placebo-controlled trial. *Acta Psychiatrica Scandinavica, 100*(1), 62–66.

Lipton, R. I. (1994). The effect of moderate alcohol use on the relationship between stress and depression. *American Journal of Public Health, 84*(12), 1913–1917.

Livesley, W., Jang, K. L., & Vernon, P. A. (1998). Phenotypic and genetic structure of traits delineating personality disorder. *Archives of General Psychiatry, 55*(10), 941–948.

Luo, H., Meng, F., Jia, Y., & Zhao, X. (1998). Clinical research on the therapeutic effect of electroacupuncture treatment in patients with depression. *Psychiatry and Clinical Neuroscience, 52*, S338–S340.

Malhi, G. S., Lagopoulos, J., Ward, P. B., Kumari, V., Mitchell, P. B., Parker, G. B., et al. (2004). Cognitive generation of affect in bipolar depression: an fMRI study. *European Journal of Neuroscience, 19*(3), 741–754.

Mapother, E. (1926). Discussion on manic–depressive psychosis. *British Medical Journal, 2,* 872–879.

Matussek, P., Soeldner, M. L., & Nagel, D. (1982). Neurotic depression: results of cluster analysis. *Journal of Nervous & Mental Disease, 170*(10), 588–597.

McCrae, R. R., & Costa, P. T. (1985). Updating Norman's 'adequacy taxonomy': intelligence and personality dimensions in natural language questionnaires. *Journal of Personality and Social Psychology, 49,* 710–721.

McCullough Jr., J. P. (2000). *Treatment for chronic depression. Cognitive behavioural analysis system of psychotherapy (CBASP).* New York, NY: The Guilford Press.

Meltzer, H. (2004). Neuropsychopharmacology in the media: did they get it right? *CINP newsletter,* 1–18.

Miller, W. R., & Rollnick, S. (1991). *Motivational interviewing: preparing people to change addictive behaviour.* New York, NY: The Guilford Press.

Millon, T., & Davis, R. O. (1996). *Disorders of personality: DSM-IV and beyond* (2nd ed.). New York, NY: John Wiley & Sons.

Minter, R. E., & Mandel, M. R. (1979). The treatment of psychotic major depressive disorder with drugs and electroconvulsive therapy. *Journal of Nervous & Mental Disease, 167,* 726–733.

Mitchell, P. B., Parker, G. B., Gladstone, G. L., Wilhelm, K., & Austin, M.-P. V. (2003). Severity of stressful life events in first and subsequent episodes of depression: the relevance of depressive subtype. *Journal of Affective Disorders, 73*(3), 245–252.

Mitchell, P., Malhi, G., Redwood, B. L., & Ball, J. (2004). *Australian and New Zealand clinical practice guideline for the treatment of bipolar disorder. Australia and New Zealand Journal of Psychiatry, 38,* 280–305. Canberra: Commonwealth Department of Health and Aged Care.

Nemets, B., Stahl, Z., & Belmaker, R. H. (2002). Addition of omega-3 fatty acid to maintenance medication treatment for recurrent unipolar depressive disorder. *American Journal of Psychiatry, 159*(3), 477–479.

Parker, G. (1983). *Parental overprotection. A risk factor in psychosocial development.* London: Grune and Stratton, Inc.

Parker, G. (2001). 'New' and 'old' antidepressants: all equal in the eyes of the lore? *British Journal of Psychiatry, 179,* 95–96.

Parker, G. (2004). *Dealing with depression. A common sense guide to mood disorders.* Sydney: Allen & Unwin. 2nd Ed.

Parker, G. (2004). Evaluating treatments for the mood disorders: time for the evidence to get real. *Australian & New Zealand Journal of Psychiatry, 38*(6), 408–414.

Parker, G. (2005). Beyond major depression. *Psychological Medicine, 35,* 467–474.

Parker, G., & Gladstone, G. (2004). Capacity of the 10-item depression in the medically ill screening measure to detect depression 'caseness' in psychiatric out-patients. *Psychiatry Research, 127,* 283–287.

Parker, G., & Hadzi-Pavlovic, D. (1984). Modification of levels of depression in mother-bereaved women by parental and marital relationships. *Psychological Medicine, 14*(1), 125–135.

Parker, G., & Hadzi-Pavlovic, D. (Eds). (1996). *Melancholia: a disorder of movement and mood. A phenomenological and neurobiological review.* New York, NY: Cambridge University Press.

Parker, G., & Malhi, G. (2001). Are atypical antipsychotic drugs also atypical antidepressants? *Australian & New Zealand Journal of Psychiatry, 35*, 631–638.

Parker, G., & Parker, K. (2003). Which antidepressants flick the switch? A review. *Australian & New Zealand Journal of Psychiatry, 37*, 464–468.

Parker, G., & Roy, K. (2002). Examining the utility of a temperament model for modeling non-melancholic depression. *Acta Psychiatrica Scandinavica, 106*(1), 54–61.

Parker, G., Roy, K., Hadzi-Pavlovic, D., & Pedic, F. (1992). Psychotic (delusional) depression: a meta-analysis of physical treatments. *Journal of Affective Disorders, 24*(1), 17–24.

Parker, G., Hadzi-Pavlovic, D., Roussos, J., Wilhelm, K., Mitchell, P., Austin, M. P., et al. (1998a). Non-melancholic depression: the contribution of personality, anxiety and life events to subclassification. *Psychological Medicine, 28*(5), 1209–1219.

Parker, G., Gladstone, G., Roussos, J., Wilhelm, K., Mitchell, P., Hadzi-Pavlovic, D., et al. (1998b). Qualitative and quantitative analyses of a 'lock and key' hypothesis of depression. *Psychological Medicine, 28*(6), 1263–1273.

Parker, G., Gladstone, G., Mitchell, P., Wilhelm, K., & Roy, K. (2000). Do early adverse experiences establish a cognitive vulnerability to depression on exposure to mirroring life events in adulthood? *Journal of Affective Disorders, 57*(1–3), 209–215.

Parker, G., Hilton, T., Bains, J., & Hadzi-Pavlovic, D. (2001a). Cognitive-based measures screening for depression in the medically ill: the DMI-10 and DMI-18. *Acta Psychiatrica Scandinavica, 105*(6), 419–426.

Parker, G., Hilton, T., Hadzi-Pavlovic, D., & Bains, J. (2001b). Screening for depression in the medically ill: the suggested utility of a cognitive-based approach. *Australian & New Zealand Journal of Psychiatry, 35*, 474–480.

Parker, G., Hilton, T., Hadzi-Pavlovic, D., & Irvine, P. (2001c). Clinical and personality correlates of a new measure of depression: a general practice study. *Australian & New Zealand Journal of Psychiatry, 37*(1), 104–109.

Parker, G., Roy, K., Mitchell, P., Wilhelm, K., Malhi, G., & Hadzi-Pavlovic, D. (2002a). Atypical depression: a reappraisal. *American Journal of Psychiatry, 159*(9), 1480–1481.

Parker, G., Both, L., Olley, A., Hadzi-Pavlovic, D., Irvine, P., & Jacobs, G. (2002b). Defining disordered personality functioning. *Journal of Personality Disorders, 16*(6), 503–522.

Parker, G., Anderson, I. M., & Haddad, P. (2003a). Clinical trials of antidepressant medications are producing meaningless results. *British Journal of Psychiatry, 183*(2), 102–104.

Parker, G., Roy, K., & Eyers, K. (2003b). Cognitive behavior therapy for depression? Choose horses for courses. *American Journal of Psychiatry, 160*(5), 825–834.

Parker, G., Parker, K., Malhi, G., Wilhelm, K., & Mitchell, P. (2004). Studying personality characteristics in bipolar depressed subjects: how comparator group selection can dictate results. *Acta Psychiatrica Scandinavica, 109*(5), 376–382.

Parker, G., Brotchie, H., & Parker, K. (2005). Is combination olanzapine and antidepressant medication associated with more rapid movement in depression than use of antidepressant alone? *The American Journal of Psychiatry, 162*, 796–798.

Paykel, E. S. (1971). Classification of depressed patients: a cluster analysis derived grouping. *British Journal of Psychiatry, 118*(544), 275–288.

Peet, M. (2003). Eicosapentaenoic acid in the treatment of schizophrenia and depression: rationale and preliminary double-blind clinical trial results. *Prostaglandins Leukotrienes & Essential Fatty Acids, 69*(6), 477–485.

Quinton, D., & Rutter, M. (1984). Parenting behaviour of mothers raised 'In Care'. In A. R. Nicol (Ed.), *Longitudinal studies in child psychology and psychiatry: practical lessons from research experience.* Chichester: Wiley Press.

Robinson, L. A., Berman, J. S., & Neimeyer, R. A. (1990). Psychotherapy for the treatment of depression: a comprehensive review of controlled outcome research. *Psychological Bulletin, 108*, 30–49.

Rodgers, B., Korten, A. E., Jorm, A. F., Jacomb, P. A., Christensen, H., & Henderson, A. S. (2000). Non-linear relationships in associations of depression and anxiety with alcohol use. *Psychological Medicine, 30*(2), 421–432.

Rutter, M. (1987). Temperament, personality, and personality disorder. *British Journal of Psychiatry, 150*, 443–458.

Sachs, G. S., Koslow, C. L., & Ghaemia, S. N. (2000). The treatment of bipolar depression. *Bipolar Disorders, 2*, 726–733.

Segal, Z. V., Williams, J. M. G., & Teasdale, J. (2002). *Mindfulness-based cognitive therapy for depression. A new approach to preventing relapse.* New York, NY: The Guilford Press.

Seligman, M. E. (1972). Learned helplessness. *Annual Review of Medicine*, 207–412.

Seligman, M. E. (1975). *Helplessness. On depression, development, and death.* San Francisco, CA: WH Freeman and Company.

Shahar, G., Blatt, S. J., Zuroff, D. C., & Pilkonis, P. A. (2003). Role of perfectionism and personality disorder features in response to brief treatment for depression. *Journal of Consulting & Clinical Psychology, 71*(3), 629–633.

Singh, N. A., Clements, K. M., & Fiatarone Singh, M. A. (2001). The efficacy of exercise as a long-term antidepressant in elderly subjects: a randomized, controlled trial. *Journals of Gerontology: Series A: Biological Sciences & Medical Sciences, 56A*(8), M497–M504.

Spiker, D. G., Weiss, J., Dealy, R., Griffin, S., Hanin, I., Neil, J., et al. (1985). The pharmacological treatment of delusional depression. *American Journal of Psychiatry, 142*(4), 430–436.

Stoll, A. L., Severus, E., Freeman, M. P., Rueter, S., Zboyan, H. A., Diamond, E., et al. (1999). Omega 3 fatty acids in bipolar disorder: preliminary double-blind, placebo-controlled trial. *Archives of General Psychiatry, 56*(5), 407–412.

Stuart, S., & Robertson, M. (2003). *Interpersonal psychotherapy: a clinician's guide.* London: Oxford University Press.

Svrakic, D. M., Whitehead, C., Przybeck, T. R., & Cloninger, C. (1993). Differential diagnosis of personality disorders by the seven-factor model of temperament and character. *Archives of General Psychiatry, 50*(12), 991–999.

Terman, M., & Terman, J. S. (1995). Treatment of seasonal affective disorder with high-output negative ionizer. *Journal of Alternative and Complementary Medicine, 1*, 87–92.

Terman, M., Terman, J. S., & Ross, D. C. (1998). A controlled trial of timed bright light and negative air ionization for treatment of winter depression. *Archives of General Psychiatry, 55*(10), 875–882.

Vollrath, M., Alnaes, R., & Torgersen, S. (1998). Coping styles predict change in personality disorders. *Journal of Personality Disorders, 12*(3), 198–209.

Walsh, B. T., Seidman, S. N., Sysko, R., & Gould, M. (2002). Placebo response in studies of major depression: variable, substantial, and growing. *Journal of the American Medical Association, 287*(14), 1840–1847.

Widiger, T. A. (1998). Four out of five ain't bad. *Archives of General Psychiatry, 55*(10), 865–866.

Williams Jr., J. W., Mulrow, C. D., Chiquette, E., Noel, P. H., Aguilar, C., & Cornell, J. (2000). A systematic review of newer pharmacotherapies for depression in adults: evidence report summary. *Annals of Internal Medicine, 132*(9), 743–756.

Winokur, G. (1991). *Mania and depression. A classification of syndrome and disease.* Baltimore, MD: John Hopkins University Press.

World Health Organization. (1992). *ICD-10. The ICD-10 classification of mental and behavioral disorders' clinical descriptions and diagnostics guidelines* (10th ed., revised). Geneva: World Health Organization.

World Health Organization. (1997). *Composite International Diagnostic Interview 2.1. CIDI Interview Manual.*

Zuroff, D. C., Blatt, S. J., Sotsky, S. M., Krupnick, J. L., Martin, D. J., Sanislow III, C. A., et al. (2000). Relation of therapeutic alliance and perfectionism to outcome in brief outpatient treatment of depression. *Journal of Consulting & Clinical Psychology, 68*(1), 114–124.

Index

Page numbers in *italics* refer to the words extracted from tables and figures.